Menopause
35 Women Speak

CAROLINE VOLLANS

Remembering my great aunt
Agnes Freeman
whose story was never heard

CONTENTS

INTRODUCTION

Menopause, a natural stage in every woman's life, remains something of a taboo subject. It is not so long ago that menopausal women were seen as mad – the mad woman (not) in the attic. Social perceptions of the menopause are often shrouded in silence, embarrassment and even shame. Euphemisms are used rather than declaring the word. The M-word does not sit comfortably in everyday vernacular.

The flip side of the coin is that the typical symptoms of the menopause get overexposure. Hot flushes, mood swings, and a lack of sexual libido are all liberally joked about, by women and men. This is menopause as cliché: the same old material vacuously repeated, sabotaging a broader and more nuanced knowledge and understanding. Humour can be helpful to some women some of the time, but if we only hear about the menopause as light entertainment, we neglect a serious and necessary engagement with it.

Notwithstanding these points, the menopause is now getting increased exposure of a thoughtful and considered nature. Radio 4's *Woman's Hour* gives substantial air time to exploring its various facets; ITV's *Loose Women* regularly broadcasts frank conversations; Meg Mathews aims at taking the taboo out of the menopause on her website; Mariella Frostrup shares her journey in *The Truth about the Menopause* (BBC 1, November 2018); Radio 4's *Start the Week* (November 2018) considers whether Marie-Antoinette's heavy vaginal bleeding was the onset of uterine cancer or premature menopause;

BBC 3's *Fleabag* includes a scene of an older woman sharing with a younger woman the horrors and delights of her menopause; BBC1's *Countryfile Spring Diaries* (May 2019) features women swimming in ice cold water to ease their symptoms and Radio 4's *The Archers* (June 2020) tells us about Kate, a forty-two year old woman, coming to terms with her early menopause.

Advertising, too, brings the menopause to our attention. From the daily papers to the sides of buses a plethora of products and treatments are displayed, all claiming to make it less troublesome. Images of women blossoming due to hormone treatments or nutritional supplements are a familiar sight, and new lines of clothing which claim to put an end to night sweats have found their way to billboards on the High Street and London Underground.

Menopause cafes and support groups offer spaces for women to get together and help each other. Women in Sport researches the benefits of exercise and organises groups providing opportunities for women to be active. There is an annual World Menopause Day aimed at raising awareness of women's mid-life health and well-being. The British Menopause Society (BMS) is working with healthcare professionals up and down the country to increase their knowledge and expertise. Research tells us that more employers are putting menopause awareness and support on their radar.

Menopause, then, is clearly on the map beyond the realms of light entertainment. Despite all of this, the most commonly used phrase during my research was 'the menopause is still not talked about'. Many women felt strongly, if not militantly about this. *Menopause: 35 Women Speak* is a response to this.

It was striking to hear just how keen women were to get involved and share their experiences and thoughts in the hope that it might be helpful to their contemporaries and future generations. Word got around – one woman led to another woman, led to a friend, led to a friend of a friend, led to a work colleague, led to another colleague overseas, and on it went. This is something that seems to happen among women. I also joined women attending community Menopause support groups, GP-run groups and Menopause cafes. This enabled *Menopause: 35 Women Speak* to represent women from a range of social and ethnic backgrounds: it is not exclusively the stories of the white, professional, middle-class in London.

All contributors were asked to respond to just one question:

What would you like to say about the menopause?

The intention of an open-ended question was to avoid the prompts and presumptions implicit in a questionnaire – I wanted more of a free-association approach. Consequently, the women openly share their anecdotes, raise questions, raise further questions, detail their confusions and conflicts, manifest deep emotion and express their innermost thoughts and feelings about what it is to be a woman at this time of her life.

Each woman participates in one of three ways; speech, writing or art. There was just one limit – a maximum of twenty minutes for spoken contributions. At the outset, I intended to leave in all speech mannerisms and idiosyncrasies, but my ideas about this changed - reading directly transcribed speech can not only be difficult, but is not much fun either. More importantly, it can involve a preoccupation with the mechanics of the speech rather than the content. Consequently, I edited the transcripts (as little as possible) to avoid this. All written pieces and artwork have been untouched.

Several common threads arose throughout the book - the main one being that the menopause is unspoken, uncertain and unknown about. What is it to be perimenopausal? How do these symptoms differ from menopausal ones, if they do? What happens when the menopause ends? How do we know it has ended? Do various feelings and states of mind originate from the effects of the menopause, or are they also to do with the more general process of ageing and other factors that occur in the middle years? Is Hormone Replacement Therapy (HRT) a viable and safe option? These are just some of the questions and uncertainties that can flummox and perplex women.

A salient feature of this collection is the polarisation of women's experiences. What is felt as a loss for one woman is a gain for the next; some women want to hold onto their periods, others can't wait to get rid of them; some women enjoy a certain freedom that comes with invisibility, others do all they can to remain noticed; some women welcome the process of ageing and the beginning of a new era in life, others resist it; some women celebrate getting older, others mourn the loss of their youth; and some women feel aspects of all these things.

Menopause: 35 Women Speak is not arranged into themed chapters: this would involve trying to fit women's experiences neatly into categories. Menopause is too complicated and messy for this. Despite some inevitable overlaps, each woman's experience is unique – every woman speaks from her singular, subjective place. It is this particularity that is paramount in this book. There is no such thing as an archetypal menopause, there is no such thing as an archetypal woman.

In all, the menopause is a multi-faceted physiological and psychological terrain that can be tricky, if not incredibly wearing and painful, to navigate. For some women, their menopause is a nightmare, for others it goes almost unnoticed and for the majority it is somewhere between the two.

Working closely with so many women has been enlightening, moving, sometimes funny and always humbling for me. Most of all, it has been my great pleasure to work with each of these women, who were willing and brave enough to share their stories, and most of whom I would never otherwise have encountered. A wonderful tapestry has been the outcome.

I thank you all.

JAYNE

I woke up in the morning, hadn't had a period for months, and all I can say is I felt like Britt Ekland in The Wicker Man. I felt … I felt beautiful. I was on some crazy hormonal one where I chucked on a seventies dress at nine in the morning, chucked my hair up and we went off for the day.

So, I was thinking about kind of mourning at the loss of being yourself, and acceptance of that. And, I guess, from that it made me think about how my menopause just crept up on me. I look back now, quite a few years, and I think things first started changing, like really sleepless nights and sweating at night, that I didn't really link with perimenopause – that must have been knocking ten years ago.

I then gently became aware that my periods were changing and, I guess, that really hit me. I've never wanted to have children – my life's gone down a different path and I don't regret my choices. Even though I could've had children but didn't, there was still something about my periods stopping that hit me on the most profound, deep level that was *serious* mourning.

I can remember having gaps of not having a period for a few months and I actually went through this whole phase of when I did get a period I *loved* it. It took my friend to remind me about how much I've moaned about my periods for the whole of my life. I sort of hated periods, but suddenly I loved them. I knew they were coming to an end – I knew things were changing and that felt *very* emotional.

I went through a whole gap of not having a period and then I had a couple of what I'd call magical periods. I suddenly came on and there was one which was *so* intense. I woke up in the morning, hadn't had a period for months, and all I can say is I felt like Britt Ekland in *The Wicker Man*. I felt ... I felt beautiful. I was on some crazy hormonal one where I chucked on a seventies dress at nine in the morning and chucked my hair up. We were going on holiday and we stopped in Avebury which is one of my favourite places. I got out of the car and said, 'I think I'm coming on', and so I had my period feeling like this just *fantastic* woman – I've never felt like it before. It was *intense*. I don't think I looked particularly fantastic – I looked like a totally mad woman. But what I felt was *gorgeous* and I had a period. I think that was probably my last one, so I felt like I'd kind of said goodbye to my periods in this wonderful, wonderful way.

I kind of accepted – that was the point of acceptance – that there was something that had shifted. It felt like I'd been allowed to kind of say goodbye. I still kind of regretted not having periods. So, first there's a deep mourning and then an acceptance starts coming in – maybe this was about the time when I wanted to get involved in setting up a group (for menopause support) and just be aware that other women were experiencing stuff too.

And, just looking at myself, other things are happening in your life if you're going through the menopause in your forties and fifties. It isn't just the physical symptoms, it's the life-changes of responsibility for parents or, if you have them, kids leaving home. So, you redress your life. There's a point where you kind of think, 'Oh my god I'm never going to fit in everything that I want to', and that's *massive*. It's just kind of *everything* – it's not the just the hot flushes, that's all absolutely bloody horrible, but it's so much more than that.

There was as a point in my life, maybe in my 30s, when I stopped referring to myself and my friends as girls and we became women. And it was like, 'Oh my god, how did that happen?', and it felt like one of those moments – suddenly I'm *not* a woman. It's like the 'Three Ages of Woman' – the Klimt picture that I've always loved. As a very young woman I loved it. And you realise you're going into that old lady category bit of it – you are no longer this youthful maiden, you know, cradling a babe. You're this kind of older woman who's going through this scientific experiment every time she looks in the mirror – this is what it feels like to me.

So, I don't know. I kind of want to embrace it, and I do embrace it and I'm totally open about menopause and I want to hear people talk about it. I don't want to wish it away because if I wish it away, I'm wishing my life away. But, yes, it's a journey, and, yes, it hits you.

I feel quite emotional at this point, so I think that's me done.

After a short pause Jayne thought of something else that was important to say:

There's something also about how people see you as a woman. I've worked with older people for years and you always say you feel the same inside, and you do. But sometimes it's a bit of a shock when you look in the mirror, especially if you're standing next to a young woman. But it's also about how other people perceive you – how people see older women.

I was once very struck by a comment from an older woman who I worked with very closely: she was one of my volunteers. She dyed her hair pink when she was in her seventies, well pink and blue. And she did it because as an older woman she felt invisible. At the time I kind of thought I got it, but the older I get the more I get it. I've never wanted particularly to conform, you know. I will still go out. I still party, I still go to gigs (not very often because I can't hack it anymore) and I refuse to be invisible.

Sometimes me and a woman mate have conversations and look at each other and what we were wearing – we must be seen totally as a mad pair of older women!

So, it's kind of the perceptions of other people of what we *should* be as women, and how we should fit in that just makes me want to *roar* at the world with frustration. I'm not having it. I will be who I will be, and I will still go for it as much as I physically can the older I get. There's a side of me that really wants to embrace my mid-life crisis, so I'll still go to gigs and I still go to festivals and, yes, I'll feel it afterwards, but I'm not going down without a fight, and I want things to change.

Women *need* to be who they are, they need to shout loudly about it.

JANE

It was a like a fairy story and that was the last time I ever saw any menstrual blood. I didn't know it was going to be the last time, but the stain looked like three jewels, so I knew it was something very special.

What I was going to say, first of all, is that I'm very interested in blood and I've written quite a lot about blood and the menopause is the cessation, as it were, of bleeding. What I liked about my periods – because I can't talk about the menopause without putting it into some context – was the fact that it was natural to bleed.

I mean if you wound yourself as a child you constantly apply plasters because bleeding, usually, is a sign that there is something wrong. I've talked to doctors about this and some people who become ophthalmologists do so because there's no blood involved, not even in surgery if they're doing it right. One of the things I have been told that surgeons fear most is finding blood in the wrong places: blood where they're not in control of it. So, my periods were important to me. I liked my periods a great deal because they were a sign of health, of being able to smell blood and I liked the smell of it. I was never fastidious, I liked bleeding. So, yes, the menopause was the cessation of bleeding.

It wasn't a bad time for me. I've had many, many worse times. Maybe the menopause and how you respond to the menopause – I haven't thought any of these things through, but just allowing myself to play – is determined to some degree by how many bad or distressing or pathological events you've had prior to the menopause, how much trauma. For some people the menopause comes as a major traumatic event – it didn't do that for me. It wasn't a bad time at all.

My daughter's fifty-one, so she's kind of perimenopausal. I think she's a little bit later than me and she keeps saying, 'Mum I don't remember the menopause as being anything you really seemed to make any fuss about.' My mother, who I wasn't close to, was bipolar, so bipolar that I'm not sure the menopause was a big issue for her. So, my daughter who I am very close to, in an unholy way, can't recall me being in any sort of drama about the menopause.

If I think about it, which I did last night, the first thought is, 'When was the last time I bled?' and that I do remember. I don't remember the date, although I could work it out. But the last time I bled I was in South London, which is a very unusual location for me, and I was in an antique kind-of reclaimed fireplace shop. I went to this little loo at the back of the shop and there were just three tiny, literally, like little emeralds, *rubies* – no they weren't emeralds, that would have been very gross – they were rubies! I don't even like emeralds. There were three tiny ruby marks, almost like stencils in my pants. I hadn't had a period for a while, though I'd obviously had menopausal symptoms. I'll come back to the one symptom that stayed with me and I don't like, but there were just these three tiny marks. It was a like a fairy story and that was the last time I ever saw any menstrual blood. I didn't know it was going to be the last time, but the stain looked like three jewels, so I knew it was something special.

In a sense, for those who get dramatic symptoms with the menopause – similar to when you have migraines or any kind of chronic physical condition – if a letter came from 'on high' telling you that on this specific day it will end, I think that would make things more tolerable. But one doesn't get such letters. I suffer from terrible IBS and have had no such letter. I did have some dramatic symptoms with the menopause, but because my life was so engaged – and I'll come back to that – it didn't really matter.

So, that was the last time I saw non-pathological blood and that's why menstrual blood was so precious to me, because it's not pathological, and so often blood does signify pathology we dread. Well, I dread it because I also have had four miscarriages. Fortunately, I ended up with two children – if I hadn't, I would have been devastated. So, I've seen a lot of blood pathologically, a lot of blood.

14

I loved my periods and I was sad when they ended. No doubt people have talked to you about whether they've taken HRT or any of those things. I took nothing. I haven't stayed in touch with the most modern developments with HRT, but personally I am very against all these hormones, and people often find they get a return of symptoms after they stop taking HRT.

For me I suppose the only remaining ... it's not an edifice, I don't know what the right word is for it – of the menopause is that my whole-body temperature has changed, and I prefer being cool to hot. Since the menopause I never ever go to a restaurant or to a social event without thinking, 'Am I going to be too warm?' I don't like being too warm. I hate being warm in a restaurant, and in bed.

Oh, when did I menopause, probably that's important? I was trying to work it out for my daughter because daughters feel these things are very important. I have a daughter and a son; my son wouldn't be interested. In fact, the subject of the menopause came up in a session only last week with someone I have been seeing professionally for a long time. We were talking about the fact he didn't know what the menopause was – I couldn't believe it. I told him to go home and talk to his wife about it, and if he was too shy then to google it – that was his homework.

I can't remember, but I was probably perimenopausal at about forty-nine and probably menopaused by about fifty-three. My whole endocrinological and hormonal system changed and now I like to be cooler than my husband. Before the menopause I liked to sleep very close to him and we had similar temperatures – we probably held each other most nights. Since I menopaused I don't like to sleep very close and, I'm afraid to say, we now have a very large eight foot bed and we sleep – something that I never ever dreamt was possible – head to toe because I just do not want a lot of covers on me and he wants a lot of covers. We have a large dog, a vizsla, who also sleeps somewhere in the middle with us – she gives forth a great deal of heat. So, there's my husband who wants to be warm, I want to be cold. I blame the menopause.

I kind of think, how did I get through the menopause so undramatically in a sense? I have talked to older women about the menopause – in the way that I've talked to younger women about post-natal depression. My own observation is that it depends whether you see the menopause as *gates of death*, symbolic death not literal death, or *gates of life*. I was fortunate because, for me, the menopause was gates of life for reasons that I can elucidate – I'll come back to that. But I think that for women, particularly when women are having children later and later, it can be very difficult because often they've given up careers in order to have children and then they have their children and their careers get left behind if they haven't been working part-time. Whereas, for me, I had my daughter when I was twenty-four and my son, because I'd had all these miscarriages and this cacophony of blood and flesh – when I was thirty-one. So, I had my children young and I was still very much evolving. In fact, I'd gone to university because I couldn't have another child. I was about thirty when I went to university and then immediately got pregnant, but that's another story.

So, by the time I got to the menopause I had just qualified as a psychoanalyst and, as you know, it takes several years to become a psychoanalyst. I'd started my analysis when I was about twenty-nine and I'd been a student counsellor at London University, but wasn't qualified as a psychoanalyst until my early forties. What got me through my menopause was passion – I had the most passionate intellectual relationship. The editor of a journal read and very much liked something I had written and asked to meet me and so we started to collaborate. I remember thinking, during the menopause, that this is the most wonderful – I can't think of the right word because it wasn't a mechanism, there was nothing mechanical about it at all, and it wasn't an artefact – whatever it was – it was an intense and meaningful relationship with another human being who taught me how to do something I'd never done before. Overnight *Fowlers English Usage* became my bible! I was utterly absorbed. I went on to co-edit two other books with female colleagues. It had never occurred to me before the menopause that I would become a writer as well as practise full-time as a psychoanalyst.

All the time I was going through these unpleasant symptoms. As I'm an insomniac the dreadful sleeplessness that so many people are struck with when they're menopausal wasn't really an affliction for me. The afflictions were really hot flushes and the heat change, bloating maybe. But what carried me through this whole period of menopause, so that I barely noticed it really, was this relationship. I learnt how to edit, I learnt how to take myself more seriously, more fastidiously as a writer. And then I went on to write my first book which was due to his mentoring.

So, the menopause timing was significant because I was going through this transitional stage into becoming a writer, learning how to edit – something which is very methodical which I'm not at all and I had to concentrate. It was like learning a new language, so I barely noticed the menopause. For many women that doesn't happen. They don't have that symmetrical happening of something completely new in their lives literally occurring when they're going through the menopause. I would lie in the bath, looking at my body and think, 'Apart from all the professional work I'm doing, this is the most wonderful device – perhaps device is the right word – for not grieving and mourning, but going forward as a writer'.

Another important feature of my experience was the Menopause Group. There were six very close girlfriends, actually to begin with it was called the 'pre-menopausal' group. We met monthly for years. We formed it as we were going into the menopause, we were at different stages. We then called it the 'post-menopausal group' and then it became, much later, the 'fractured hip' group – although, thankfully, I was not one of those unlucky people. One of the common menopausal symptoms we seemed to share which was a consolation in itself was that if you laughed or got up suddenly after you sneezed you became enuretic and you might even wet your pants. In the group we would talk about going into Waitrose and instead of buying nappies we were looking at enuretic pads! Phew, thank goodness that phase has passed, at least for me.

So many of the symptoms you experience in menopause can mask other things going on in your body. In my consulting room when I listen to what may or may not be psychosomatic symptoms and people who start bleeding after the menopause, I always think of Thomas Mann's – I don't think it can be *The White Swan*, it's *The Black Swan* – where this elderly woman thinks she's having an extraordinary erotic experience with her body and lost youth and, in fact, she's got ovarian cancer.

HILARY

Woman's Capacity (484 minus 18), 20

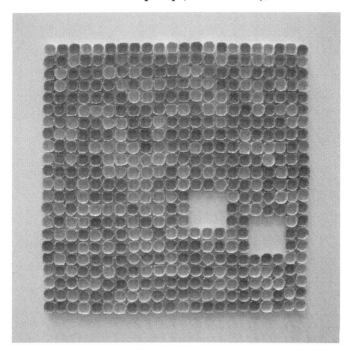

This piece is a calculation of the number of eggs actually ovulated during a woman's reproductive life, although it's probably less than this …

MAARYA

It makes me sad that in my culture it's not something that's talked about and you have to hide all of these things, just get on with it.

A cultural perspective is important for me, because when I first heard about it, I thought, 'Oh my gosh, yes, what is it? What do we call *it* in our culture? How do we describe it? Who have I heard talk about it?'

My culture is South Asian – Indian background. Obviously, all my ancestors' heritage is from India, and my parents were first generation immigrants to this country. I've never *ever* heard anyone talk about menopause. When I look back now, I think my mum was possibly going through some of the things that I'm going through, but she described it as 'how the world has changed', and 'the world isn't like what it used to be.' It's my assumption that that's what she must have meant because she and her mates or her relatives used to come and talk about how things felt different, how the world wasn't how it used to be and that was it – that was all they'd say. So, I'm making a link in thinking it could have been about menopause, but I'm not sure whether it was that or whether the world was just feeling different for them. I remember this being around the time she would have been the age I am now, approaching fifty.

But I never remember anyone saying anything about what it was or what happened. In our culture the only thing they used to say was 'It's finished' – by this *it* they meant the monthlies.' So, they'd say something like, 'Oh, yes, so-and-so is a bit older because she doesn't get it anymore.' Even the monthlies for us when we were younger were described as *it*. 'Is *it* here?' 'Has *it* gone?' Only when I got older, and I think it was after I got married, I heard the name for *it* – the period. I don't know if that's cultural or religious – I'm of the Muslim faith.

So, coming up to a certain age, I was very aware of the menopause simply because of the people I'd been around, the people I'd seen experience it and reading about it. I think reading taught me a lot – what it is, what to expect. I myself, then looked it up and read up a bit more about the science behind it and what happens. But I think going into it has been interesting for me – how I feel, my perception of it and what I'm experiencing. And for those around me too – my husband, my kids – that's been interesting, hilariously funny at times as well as really sad.

I don't officially know whether I'm in *it* – in the menopause – or if I'm going to experience something else that's going to lead me into it. I went to the doctor and she said, 'Yes, you could be,' and that was it. I've heard other people say, 'Oh, they gave me a blood test and said, 'Yes, you are menopausal'. I didn't ask for a blood test. People say they can determine whether you are or not, but I didn't really want one. I didn't really want or need a blood test to tell me things are changing; I can tell myself.

The changes have been very emotional, that's been huge. The other thing that's changed is, obviously, my monthly cycle – it's erratic. I always used to have a twenty-eight-day cycle, but now it goes up and down. It can be a fifty-six day one or a ten day one. Also, the fact of age. I'm forty-eight now and thinking, 'Yes, I will be going through it,' or 'This is the age when I should be.' I guess you prepare yourself a little bit. I think they're the three key things.

The emotional thing though – oh my goodness me! First, we've had building works going on, my husband's not been well and three children to look after. So, it's difficult to pinpoint whether all the emotional was just me, or whether it was these other factors going on around me. But, as I've kind of thought about it, I've though that it *must* be the menopause because now things are better and more settled. The kids are where they wanted to be, K's health is as good as it ever will be, but some days I'll still feel bad, more so than I ever did before. I just want to cry and then I think, 'What are you crying for?' And I don't know, I just want to cry. The kids will say to me, 'Are you going to cry?' and I say, 'No, don't say that because then I will.'

Sometimes you just want to weep, and then at other times you feel like you could tackle the world.

You think, 'Yes, I'm an older person, I'm wiser, I know a little bit more,' but then in your head you're also thinking, "I don't feel any older than when the kids were little.' So, I don't know if it's all hormone-related or if it's my perspective on how I'm feeling about where I am in life. I suppose the past couple of months have been a little bit better, but before that it got to the point where the kids were saying, 'Why don't you do something?' I was though, I was doing things. I was going out, meeting friends, we were going out as a family – but it just didn't feel like I wanted to join in many things. I just wanted to just sit there. And then I'd be thinking that I'd be quite happy sewing, quite happy gardening and I'd say to myself, 'Oh my god, that means you're turning into an old woman!' That frightened me a little bit. Even now when they say. 'What are we doing today?' I think, 'You guys go and do what you like, I'm happy here'. And they say, 'You're getting so boring in your old age, mum.' So, then it makes you question why it is that you want to sit there – I'm not fifty yet – I don't know if it's psychological or biological. I just don't know.

I don't feel negative about it, I've got to say. Like I've got a friend who wouldn't even talk about it – the M word – she wouldn't say anything about it whereas I'm not like that. It is what it is, and you are who you are.

I feel, though, it's so different for my daughters – they're able to talk about it unlike thirty years ago. They know what it is and even read up about it and suggest things to me, whereas with my mum and my aunts it was something we'd never discuss. Even with my mum now I'd never be able to say what I'm going through or explain why I feel like I do. We just don't ever talk about. It's very much dismissed. Whatever goes on you just deal with it, you don't have to keep talking about it. So, that's what it's like, whereas with my kids we're trying to change the thinking about it and perceptions about it.

Some things are funny. If I'm feeling low, my daughters will laugh about it and they've named it 'manny' – it's their word for the menopause – and they ask if it's that what's making me feel like that and I say, 'I don't know, probably it is,' and we're able to talk about it openly. I said to H, my son, 'When I say menopause to you, what do you think?' He's like twenty and he went, 'Erm, uh, err, mum … don't!' We were all round the table and just laughed. So, he couldn't pinpoint what it meant, he couldn't talk about it at all. My daughters are fine – they seem to understand and want to have a more open conversation and go off and find out more about it, so they're completely different. My husband puts everything down to it, which is really interesting. So, every time I've had a bad day at work his understanding is that it's all because of *that*. I'm like, 'It's not – I don't think it is that!' So, he gives me a wide berth sometimes, or listens to me when I'm rambling and sees it as being *all* because of that. Sometimes we will talk it through though and he'll want to know about it, what's part of it, what isn't and so on – so, yes, he engages with it. We're both very much aware that we're hitting middle-age and that things are going to be different. I think generally your outlook changes. I don't know if this is a key milestone into thinking more like that as a couple, I'm not sure.

There are the different stages of the menopause, so people have talked about the perimenopause and then you hit menopause and some people have said it goes on for ten years, and some have said it goes on a lot longer, so I don't know. The physical side of it where you don't have your monthlies – you have hot flushes. Oh my gosh, oh my gosh – I've gone through a few months with them and then off and then back on, and so on. There's nothing that I can relate them to, or anything that triggers them. But it's like this heat from the bottom of your feet and it just rises like this and you can feel it and it's like this tingle. But it's quite interesting, if I'm in a meeting I don't strip and tell everyone I'm having a moment – I just kind of suffer it. Whereas I've seen some people getting really hot and they take off their cardi and put it on the table and you'll know. I don't feel like I should, though I do at home. I just say, 'My thermostat's gone'. At the moment I'm not having any – a couple of months ago there were quite a few.

I talk about all of this with one of my sisters-in-law, but I don't say anything to the older people, and never anything to the men. Men never acknowledge it openly in our culture – my husband does, but that's privately within our relationship.

I get sad moments when the kids look at me thinking, 'You're getting older and this is what you're going through.' And I'll be like, 'No, don't.' As I'm going through the menopause, I start to feel that how we used to treat our elders is now how I am being treated. I'm getting a bit older and hitting a different stage in my life. You just kind of think, coming up to fifty with all the changes in my body and the emotions going up and down, it's quite a change. A period of change in my life. That saddens me sometimes, but there's lots to look forward to as well. So, it's not as if it saddens me just because of that, but it does seem to herald middle age for me. I used to think that people who talked about menopause were old people, but it's me now. That's the sad bit, I think.

The other sad bit is that I can't talk about it with my mum. With my girls we talk about it openly now, and if I'm still here when they're going through it, it would be lovely to feel they'd be able to talk about it with me. So, yes, it makes me sad that in my culture it's not something that's talked about and you have to hide all of these things, just get on with it.

HRT is something I'm determined not to have. All I've heard is negative stuff. I haven't read up on it, I've got to say. This is just what I've heard people say. I've not explored it at all, but I think it's a pill I don't want to take. People have said that it makes it worse, others have said there's links to cancer, some people say once you get on it you don't want to come off it, so I don't know. I've heard a couple of people say it's worked well for them, but it's not something I've looked into at all. I'm completely ignorant, to be honest though. There's this bravado among women, too, about getting through it without HRT.

I think it's just outlook for me with the whole thing. I've seen people come out of it and say it's the best they've felt ever – health-wise, fitness-wise, outlook-wise. So, I'm holding onto that. I don't know if it's because you were OK and then you go through a rough time, so then when you come out of it you feel great again.

I don't think my GP's been particularly helpful. Maybe I've not pushed it enough, though I shouldn't really have to. I don't want to push it anymore at the moment unless I feel any worse and then I would want to.

So, yes, that's me.

FILO

I don't feel the pressure of, 'Oh, I'm going into the menopause, I'm getting old,' in the way I hear my friends talking about. It's not like this for me at all – the physical aspects are a lot more pronounced than these more emotional and psychological aspects.

I think the first thing that comes to mind is the physical, what changes in a person physically. Hormones have a big impact on everybody's life, and I think women particularly are very sensitive to hormonal balance and how it varies through the monthly cycle, from a very young age.

For me, the aspect of not having my period any more related to menopause doesn't exist because I had a hysterectomy, so the changes to the physical part of my body happened involuntarily a few years ago and that triggered the changes to the hormones. I guess I started feeling the symptoms a lot sooner than I would have if I hadn't had the surgery. The fact that I no longer had my period and couldn't get pregnant wasn't the effect of menopause because I couldn't have children anyway. So, my ability to get pregnant, to have a family was not a decision that I made, nor is it related to menopause. It just happened in that way with me, so I cannot relate these symptoms to menopause.

I do have menopause symptoms – feeling uncomfortable, feeling depressed, getting migraines, heat flushes. Some of them are symptoms I had at a very young age when my periods started. They actually came back with the menopause. So, these things that I remember from being a teenager, I started having them again. It's quite pronounced.

I know exactly where I am in my hormonal cycle because I get those symptoms. They're not psychological, but physical. I know this because my body changes and I feel it.

I remember my grandmother talking about it. My mother had a bad one – a really bad menopause in all aspects – and so it's something I almost had an idea of what I would have to go through. So, it wasn't a surprise in a way, and it's something that is natural. I don't take any hormone replacement; I don't believe in taking hormones. I take hormones for my thyroid because it's dysfunctional and I need to take them, but if it was something that wasn't needed, wasn't necessary, I wouldn't take hormones to replace the changes to the natural hormones.

To be honest, I don't feel the pressure of, 'Oh, I'm going into the menopause, I'm getting old,' in the way I hear my friends talking about. It's not like this for me at all. The physical aspects are a lot more pronounced than these more emotional and psychological aspects.

I think, in a way, it's because I've always had some kind of problem related to my womb, to my ovaries, to my hormones. There's always something not one hundred per cent in my body. Before having the hysterectomy, I went through many, many years where I would haemorrhage every month up to the point where I had my period for thirty-three days – I counted. I was anaemic and then I said, 'That's it, it's enough. I'm not going to get pregnant,' and, so be it, I had the hysterectomy.

So, in a way, the physical impact of hormonal changes was always more dominant for me than the psychological or emotional. And I could say that this is still true during the menopause...

TINA WRITES

Mad Menopausal Adventures

For my seventieth birthday our adult children made one of the most treasured birthday presents I have ever received. It was in a picture frame, with a handwritten list titled, '70 Things We Got from Our Mother.' It is hanging on the wall, and I love to go and read there. Number 52 said, 'Mad Menopausal Adventures (the demise of the washing-up machine).'

Our washing-up machine had broken down. I had never really wanted one, but with young children having play-dates during that phase of life, followed by hordes of teenagers descending on us, it made sense. But now it had broken, and I was finding that washing-up and drying-up together with family and their friends was a good way of staying in touch. So, when it broke down I felt that it was a good time for it to go.

While the family were at work and school I switched it off and cut the wire embedded in the wall. The horror of the teenagers on their return from school was huge, and I was given stern lectures on the science! One did Physics 'A' level and the other Chemistry.

They have dined out on this story ever since. And, we have never had a washing-up machine since! So, I can safely tell this tale.

Although I am beyond menopausal adventures, the next might be adventures in dementia – who knows?

It's definitely best not to have a washing-up machine, just in case…

JUDI WRITES

I went into an immediate menopause at forty-nine following a total hysterectomy.

It was a shock – at first I accepted medications to ameliorate symptoms, but then got off them quickly when the information came into the news about the links to cancer.

I went from being a mild person to one who yelled at cars while driving. I lost my libido and any sense of myself as a still somewhat young middle-aged woman.

I felt so much older.

Night sweats were difficult, but after about five years, it had calmed, and I had no more physical symptoms.

PAULINE

Dunes

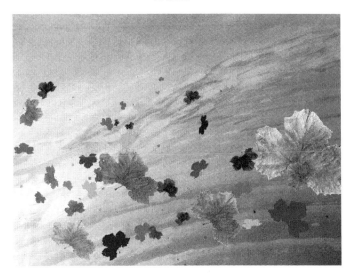

A breeze or a wind of change

over a desert sea?

GINNY

You know, some of the people that I most want to talk to in the world are older women.

The first thing I want to say is that I think it's a really good thing for people to talk about the menopause, and for you to collate lots of different experiences about it. Partly I think that because it's not that it isn't talked about now, because it is, but it's still something that's quite *unknown* about. Every medical professional you speak to seems to say something slightly different, and everybody's experience is very different, so it's a good idea to have a collated set of experiences and maybe find recurring, useful themes. And of course, it's not just a medical thing, that's the really important thing – it's like a social experience that I imagine hasn't been like this before because society hasn't been like this before. It's only in relatively recent times that large numbers of women in society have lived long enough to experience the menopause, and the fact that lots of people are experiencing it at the same time has an impact on how people see them and so on.

Apparently, it's only us and killer whales who have a menopause which is quite an exciting idea isn't it? I love the fact that killer whales have one too!

I thought I'd talk about my journey here today, actually, as an example of what it's like for me having a menopause. I came on my bike, but I've done this journey on my bike and on foot loads of times before, though not for a little while. So, I was pleased that I was coming out, it was a lovely day and I was looking forward to a cycle. And I got lost, for no reason at all. As soon as I got lost, I couldn't read – well, I could read the signposts, but I couldn't remember what they'd said thirty seconds later. As soon as that started to happen, I started to feel useless, sort of quite hot – not that real burning hot that you get at night, but quite warm – and I was just absolutely addled, I think addled is the word. So, I've just come in Mark's gate, and I got from Mark's gate to the signpost which is about ten metres away, and by the time I'd got to the signpost, even though I'd taken note that I'd come in Mark's gate, I couldn't remember which gate I'd come in. Then to compound matters I had my mobile phone with me – which I don't think helped – and it was telling me to go one way and I thought I had to go the other. The sheer amount of confusion that came out of this journey, so needlessly.

But most of the confusion came from a lack of confidence. Now I'm here, I realise that I did know the way, but I stopped so many times on the way here to check, 'Am I doing it right, am I doing it right?' For me that kind of sums up, so far, my experience of the menopause – that in the last two or three years I wouldn't say I've become more addled, but there've been more and more occasions where I've *felt* addled. And that's one of the reasons I think it's important to talk about it because I think lots of people probably feel like that. I'm sure that it's not the experience of every person, but it's quite frightening. It doesn't actually mean that you're descending into, you know, some sort of state of not knowing anything any of the time.

I've also had the experience at work, and this is another reason I think it's important to talk about it, because I think it's important to think of what the impact of having a menopause is on working women. So, I was teaching. I wasn't feeling stressed at all. I was teaching a group of six within a class of thirty. I was modelling a lesson for a less experienced teacher. I knew him, I knew the class, it was a very relaxed atmosphere. We were actually having quite a lot of fun really. It was a nice book we were reading, and the children all seemed quite happy. It wasn't a stressful situation at all. I was in the middle of a sentence and I suddenly forgot what I was saying, and then I tried to make a joke out of that. I tried to say to one of the children, 'Uh, do you know, I've forgotten where I was, can you remind where we were up to in our discussion?', which is always kind of a good teaching technique anyway to see if they're listening. And I couldn't remember the child's name. Then

I looked around the group and I couldn't remember *any* of the children's names. Then I thought I'd make contact with the teacher because I felt like I needed to check in with someone, and I said, 'Oh, Mr ...' and I couldn't remember his name either. So, everybody's names had left me. I knew where I was, I knew what I was meant to be teaching, I knew I was teaching reading, but I couldn't remember anything else. I couldn't remember *anyone's* name.

Names are probably the very worst thing for me – names and finding my way and finding directions. And, actually, that does have a knock-on effect on how you are in your career. There's a great power, especially as teachers, in knowing people's names. There's a great power, also, in being able to pull up facts and say, 'I think you'll find in such and such, that happened.' So, that's something I find hard but, of course, the more stressed you get about it – and this is true whether or not you're having the menopause – the worse it gets.

Of course, there's a bit of it that's just about life in general anyway – it's just what life's like. And I think sometimes it's really hard to know what's just life, what's just me and what's the menopause. I'm sure someone could make a very nice Venn diagram about it.

On a completely different subject, regarding the night sweats I'm utterly convinced that alcohol, especially white wine, makes night sweats worse. I think that they should do some research into that. It makes anxiety worse for me, like it'll make my heart beat really fast and I'll start worrying about all sorts of things. I'm talking about like two glasses of wine in an evening, I'm not talking about, you know, binge drinking. I will wake up in the night really, really, hot. But If I *don't* drink it's much better, and I'm quite interested to know if everybody else had had that same experience, or not. It's the sort of hot where you have to get up and press your head against the window. You know, there's that series on Netflix where the woman just stands in front of a fridge and opens the fridge door every night. Women laugh at that and say, 'Yes, that's what I feel like. That's when you have to get somewhere really cold.'

I've spoken about the negative side of it and, of course, the menopause is all about your body changing and it is a bit of a move towards ending. I think that's why it's a sad thing to think about and why it feels difficult. When you get your period at eleven, twelve or thirteen that's like a beginning of something, something to be celebrated, but your menopause feels like an end, and I think that's quite a sad feeling, in a way. I didn't realise that would make me sad …

But, also, maybe there's something positive to come out of it and I think this is one of the other reasons why it's important to talk to people. Older women, and older men as well, have an experience that young people don't have, but trying to find the positives of the menopause is hard.

Obviously not much good comes from feeling hot and confused, but the menopause is about the end of fertility and what do women offer after they are fertile? Lots! You know, some of the people I most want to talk to in the world are older women. They've got lots to offer and maybe a different view on things. I haven't, sort of, ever thought in my head or spoken to anybody about this before, but I wonder what positive things can come out of the menopause for people?

You know that idea of the 'grandmother art-therapist'? Well, that's the phrase that comes to mind for me. My relationship with my grandma was really important. So, it's that kind of moving to an older person way of being. I'm not saying that as soon as we have a menopause we have to become grandmothers either, but maybe that grandmotherly-type relationship to the world.

One positive that comes out of it is that it's much easier to talk to young people – you don't attract attention in the same way. You know, you can kind of go out looking however you want, and it's alright. Nobody really takes a great deal of notice, and there's a certain freedom in that, I suppose. So those are positives as an individual.

But, yes, I wonder what menopausal women have to offer? I think that's an important question that I don't have an answer to. But I think there is something.

ESTHER

Women like me who had children when they were older have a very different set-up of where they are likely to be in their life when they have their menopause.

One of the things I've been thinking about in relation to this is that, in a way, the whole story starts when your periods start – this is the beginning of the story, before we progress towards the end of the story. Although, of course, it's not the end of the story.

I think there is something about how times have changed. For example, my mother didn't *ever* speak to me about periods and found the whole subject matter of periods and sex or anything like that very, very difficult to talk about. I think that came out of the post-war world period and, maybe, particularly for her because she was illegitimate. She and her sister had different fathers and they didn't know who their fathers were. There was so much shame around that, you know, that made their mother's life very, very difficult socially. And the war only added to that. So, there's definitely a massive difference in contexts for women of that generation, women of my generation and then what it will be like for our children's generation.

My first period was a very lonely sort of experience, and one thing I was really struck by is that I came out of that experience with a longing or sort of ambition that when I had daughters I'd talk to them as much as they wanted about periods. And, actually, to celebrate the beginning of that phase of life. Then, of course, when it came to it my daughter was *horrified* by the idea of talking about it, and certainly of celebrating it! So, it was quite a difficult negotiation – working out what were my needs and desires and trying to match them up with what my daughter wanted and with what she was experiencing. In the end we found our way through it, and it was better than it had been when I was a child. I bought her a red suitcase and put all sorts of nice things in it including sanitary towels and stuff like that – that worked for both of us in a way.

I'm perimenopausal, so my periods are few and far between, very unpredictable – maybe once every few months or something like that. It's been going like that for a few years. Another thing that really struck me was that when my eldest daughter had her first period, I got *my* period. I think it was that thing of women living together and the hormones of other women sort of acting on you, and I just thought – *is* that really a thing? Does that happen to other parents with their first or with any of their

43

daughters? It just hadn't occurred to me. In a way I shared her first period with her because I had mine as well. I really noticed it because of them being so infrequent. I think it was definitely brought on by her hormones, so that's quite extraordinary. I think these things act on us in ways that are deeper than we sometimes recognise.

And then, not very long after that, the night before my youngest daughter's tenth birthday, again, I got my period during that night. I had really, really strong period pains all night. I generally don't get period pain – my periods have always been quite light and unnoticeable – so it was quite a big thing to have this kind of memory of her birth in my body coming out on the tenth anniversary of when I would have been in labour with her.

My mum's a little bit more forthcoming about menopause now, partly because she has dementia and so there's a lot more of her that's accessible. She's very much in the past and more prepared to talk about the past. There's a lot more available and a lot more to find out. But also, I think she *had* to talk about menopause because it seemed to be quite a strong experience for her. I'm not sure of the details of it except that her hair fell out – like *all* her hair fell out. It was almost like she was going through chemotherapy or something like that. I'm not quite sure how old she was, but in her fifties, I think.

When I was growing up my mum's hair was a very prominent feature – she had almost afro hair, so a lot of curly black hair. I think she found it quite difficult having hair like that. But when it all fell out she decided to get a wig, none of which she told us about. She lived in France at the time and we turned up and there she was with this wig. She chose the sort of hair that, in her fantasies, she would always have had which was a blond, straight bob. So, that was quite strange that she took the opportunity to re-invent herself and become quite different. It was really quite a *big* difference her having that hair – there was this outward sign, so she had to say something about it. Largely, though, it was still this very, very private thing. I think it seems that it was related to the skin condition psoriasis that her hair fell out – she had that on her scalp. I have it on my nails. I think she got frustrated because the doctors refused to see any hormonal connection between her skin condition and her menopause. It's very weird that they didn't. No-one really understands psoriasis, so why *wouldn't* it be related to hormonal changes?

I guess the other thing I'm aware of is that 'women of my generation' – women like me who had children when they were older – have a very different set-up of where they are likely to be in their life when they have their menopause. That kind of sandwich generation thing is quite particular, isn't it? I guess just the fact that my perimenopausal time coincided with my daughter's first period wouldn't have happened if I'd had children when I was younger. But also, I have ageing parents who are frail and require me to be much more proactive in the relationship. They've never been able to look after the children or anything like that, so all those relationships are very different when you have children later in life.

Hopefully, the menopause won't be too bad because I'll have an awful lot else on my plate over the next decade, potentially. Children doing exams and parents becoming older and frailer and more demanding in a certain sort of way.

I don't think that I've particularly experienced any strong effects so far in terms of symptoms. I've occasionally had hot flushes, but they're usually brought on by situations that are a bit more – I don't know – like if I've had to do a presentation or something I notice that I can get more hot and bothered and it doesn't go away as quickly. So, *if* that's what it is, it's quite subtle. Who knows what's to come in that respect? Whilst I sort of long for a context for the process of ageing, I do also think it is there and more available to us than it used to be for previous generations. I think that women are much more aware of how important their friendships are. It seems to me that all those connections you make with people when you have children bear fruit and offer support and opportunities that I don't think my mum had in the same way, probably.

I have just turned fifty, and I think that my mid-life crisis was to become a Buddhist – it could have been a lot worse! It seemed to me to be quite a positive way to have a mid-life crisis, so far anyway. It's been a big change, but I think it's brought a lot actually to my relationship with my husband and with my children. As well as that, I think that the sort of awareness, particularly the sort of body awareness and meditation and all the stuff that you do in the Buddhist practice, is probably going to be very helpful for the times that are to come.

Thinking about long term relationships and sexual identity, I think they're a bit of a mystery anyway. I don't suppose any of us really know what other people's relationships are like. Yes, you have children – we don't have the luxury of a particularly big house or anything, so we don't get that much privacy – so your sexual relationship and those things change a lot over time anyway. I don't know, I can imagine the sense of loss of being a sexual being can happen, but I can't really identify with that or with it necessarily being a problem.

Not sure what else to say except that the thing that really struck me when you mentioned doing this book was, '*Yes, I want to talk about that*'. I think that's the thing. I have a feeling there is more to my experience of it, it's just that I haven't explored it.

I'm in a little study group with three other women at the Buddhist centre which is a thing that people often do in that sort of context. It's really quite recent that we've started doing it, but it feels a bit like a women's circle or something. They've all got grown up children, my children are the youngest and we range in age between … I don't know… one of them is nearly seventy. They were quite excited about the idea of talking about the menopause, so that feels like potentially quite a good place to explore it further.

I don't have an experience of it as a medical thing yet, but I know that one of the women in that group is a GP and she's on HRT. She found it a very difficult decision to make to go on it, she was really scared because of the breast cancer link. So, even for a GP there's an awful lot of unknowns in doing something like that.

HUMA WRITES

I'm forty-five and told that I'm pre-menopausal. Three years ago, I started getting heavy periods so had to start wearing extra thick pads. I was passing huge clots and changing towels hourly. I was totally drained.

One day blood just flowed out of me, so I went to A&E. They gave me a blood transfusion, sent me home and said go to and see my GP.

I have since been referred to gynaecologists who took out two polyps. I still bleed randomly, with no particular pattern. It's not been as heavy recently, but I live life in a state of paranoia.

I sweat all day long, when everyone else is cold. In the night my bed gets soaked, and I'm sometimes changing the sheets three times a week. I feel dirty all the time, some days taking three showers.

But they have discharged me now giving me tablets – two Noriday daily. I was told this was normal and nothing to worry about.

All I want is a hysterectomy, but apparently, I'm too young. I can't afford to go privately, so I live miserably.

TATIANA

Clematis

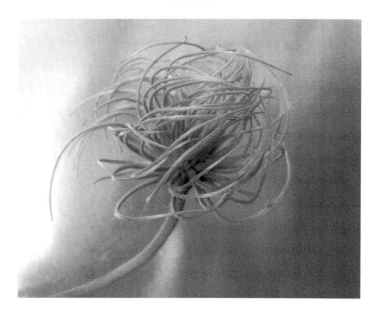

This flower has already lost all its petals and there is no pollen left, but it is not the time to give up. It's curled its stamens into an impressive whirl and stands proudly among flatly spread, brighter (younger) flowers and vibrant foliage, refusing to surrender its position. Just being there as a statement that real beauty has different dimensions.

LARA

Thinking about my period and menstruation – I don't even like saying menstruation. I don't like saying menopause – all of that stuff makes me feel a bit jealous of men.

I've been thinking so much about this and was going to write some notes, but then I thought that might make it formulaic. So, I'm just going to let myself think.

I'm fifty-one. I'm still getting my periods, but definitely, you know, perimenopausal. I get, or I got, really quite extreme night sweats. But I've changed my diet. I was telling K this morning, 'Change your diet' because my night sweats have practically stopped. Apart from Saturdays, which is why I'm eating cake today! The rest of the week I don't eat carbs or processed sugar, and I've cut down my coffee and I don't drink much alcohol. Saturday's my day off: I have coffee, alcohol, the whole lot. I rarely get night sweats anymore.

I'm also very physically, not *very* but *quite*, fit. I do a lot of running – probably about thirty miles every week. So, as a physical thing, I wouldn't say that the menopause has been, so far, in the perimenopausal stage, a massive problem for me.

But I recently went to get a smear test and I was telling the nurse, who was post-menopausal and probably sixty-something, 'God, you know, I can't wait to get my bloody menopause. I can't wait to stop my fucking periods!' She looked at me and said, 'You won't say that when it happens. It's dreadful.' I kind of laughed, and she said, 'You won't even find it funny. You'll long for your periods to come back.' And I said, 'I won't, I won't. I've never enjoyed having my periods.'

That said, I'm the kind of person who doesn't even know when I've got my period. I literally forget it's coming and then, when it arrives, I forget I've got it. So, I'll stick a tampon in, and I might only remember to change it eight hours later. I've never really had pain from my periods. I've sometimes had a bit of back pain, but the older I've got and the more physically fit I've got, the less that's bothered me. So, I've noticed my fitness and my diet have massively affected how I've felt.

The only thing I'll miss about my periods is the fact that – and I was thinking, as a feminist should I tell people this, but I do think it's quite funny – my partner, J, who is a man, right from very early on in our relationship, would get really annoyed with the fact that I would go out without any tampons and then my period would start. I would think, 'Oh, shit, my period's started,' as if every month was another surprise. He'd be like, 'I can't understand how you can be so disorganised,' and I'd say, 'It's just not a priority in my life.' It's something that, you know, irritates me and so I don't really apply myself to thinking about it.

So, J started counting the days between my periods. I don't know if he did that without me knowing, I think initially it was without me knowing. But once he'd got a pattern, he started saying to me, 'By the way, you're going to get your period in a couple of days.' At the beginning it *really* annoyed me. I thought, 'This bloody man is like taking control of my life', but actually I've become totally dependent on it and it's really useful. So, this morning I said to him as I left, 'Oh god, when's my period due?' He said, 'It should be in the next two to three days.' So, I put a tampon in my handy boiler suit pocket here.

I remember telling the nurse, 'The thing I will miss is this hilarious relationship I have with my partner, who tells me when I'm going to be getting my period.' I find it really funny, but I don't know how I survived before he was around because I never had any fucking tampons and I was endlessly having to throw knickers away because I would, you know, end up with blood in my pants.

The other side of this is that I don't have children. I've got friends who've said they've been really upset when their period ended because it's the end of being a woman and being fertile. I just don't feel that. I just feel it's an irritation that gets in the way. It's just a pain in the arse that I have to think about, and I have to buy extra stuff from the shops to look after it. I don't feel any desire to have children. I don't feel any kind of fertility or infertility thing. It doesn't boost my notion of being a woman or not. I can't wait for my periods to end.

In fact, since I've been in my mid-forties, every month I'm thinking, 'Oh, god, I really hope this month my period doesn't come.' And then it comes and I'm disappointed. It's sort of the opposite of people who want to have a baby. They're hoping their period won't start and then it starts; I'm hoping it won't come back and it keeps on fucking coming back. It just won't go away.

The other thing that has struck me is that I have very strong memories from when I was growing up of my mother having a really bad time of it with her menopause. She hasn't said this, but my memories are of her going through some quite bad stuff, being on HRT, being quite unhappy and finding it all incredibly difficult and fanning herself, and all that sort of thing. I sometimes see women at a party standing in the corner and doing that fanning, and I think of my mother over-heating and being really stressed out. This is a terrible thing to admit in a way, but I find myself feeling quite annoyed about it. I have such mixed feelings about it because when I grew up my mum used to talk about her period as 'the curse'. So, there was the curse and then there was the menopause. That word – it's such an ugly word.

So, OK, first, it's all this blood, the time of the month, the whole thing that you should be having children. Then, you're coming round to the menopause and apparently, it's this thing that makes you go a bit nuts. I Googled the word before I came to see you and I noticed many references to mood swings and irrational behaviour in middle-aged women. But, you know, I am somebody who has quite erratic behaviour anyway. I am very spontaneous; I can lose my temper and get very angry. I've been like that my whole life. It's not like suddenly I hit forty-five, got hot sweats and went a bit nuts. If anything, I feel like I've become more balanced which could be to do with a whole load of things. But this idea of women being neurotic and hysterical and unable to control their moods because of the menopause – well, that's just not my experience.

It seems to me that there's been this narrative around the menopause, certainly in the life I've had. This is why your book seems so extraordinary, precisely because so little is said about the subject. It feels like this dirty secret that women have.

My friend K said to me today that she feels dirty because she can't control her bleeding, so she's constantly having to shower. You wake up in the morning, you've been sweating all night and you wake up feeling dirty. You've got to have another shower, you've got to change the sheets, you feel bad about your partner because the bed's so wet – it's almost like you've wet your knickers. It's the feeling that you do not have control of your body. I think that's partly why I do a lot of running and why I have changed my diet, it has allowed me to take some sort of control.

The other side of the whole menopause is that it's something I'm really looking forward to. When I turned fifty a year ago, that felt like a real moment of liberation because fifty is so certainly middle-aged, so certainly no longer young. The menopause is part of that. When my periods stop, I'm going to have a fucking party. I cannot wait for the thing to end. I will celebrate.

I have had times in my life when I have wished I could pay to have a hysterectomy. That's how much I'd love to end my periods. They've been a burden, particularly when I was working as a foreign correspondent and going into areas where you wouldn't be able to find sanitary towels. I don't mean in cities, but you'd be going into places where there were wars and it wouldn't be easy to come across a sanitary towel, let alone a fucking tampon. Having a period was just a pain in the arse. I'd go into these places with dollar bills hidden in my bra and I'd have tampons all over the place, stuffed into every single pocket so that I wouldn't get caught short. So, for that to end just seemed wonderful, blissful.

I've found myself more recently thinking, 'Does this mean I'm a bit jealous of men because men don't have any of this stuff to deal with?' I've thought a lot about the whole trans movement and in the last five years I have thought much more beyond the binary. Up until my mid-forties I was stuck in binary ways of thinking around gender.

Thinking about my period and menstruation – I don't even like saying menstruation, I don't like saying menopause – and all that stuff makes me feel a bit jealous of men. OK, they get an erection and I guess it can be a bit tough when you're a teenager walking around with a sort of stick poking out of your trousers. I'm sure if you're a fifteen-year-old boy that can be quite difficult. But it's not bleeding into your fucking knickers, is it? It's not that bad. You know, you put your hand over your trousers, and it goes away. It's not like you're going to end up with blood everywhere.

When I've spoken to female friends who have real problems with heavy bleeding, which I've never had so far, touch wood, I think it's a real restriction on their freedom. It can create a fear of going out. You don't want to go out wearing fucking nappies in case you end up with blood all over the place. But once the blood starts flowing you can't stop it. I resent that, I really resent it. Maybe I feel a bit resentful of being a woman.

But, you know, when I raise the whole trans stuff, it's not like I've got some secret trans desire to become a man – that isn't what I feel at all. I'm very happy being a woman. I think being a woman's great. I like being part of an idea of sisterhood, even though I don't think sisterhood exists. I really like other women, women have inspired me, and I'm lucky to be with a man who's a feminist and to know a lot of men who are feminists. I don't want to be a man; I don't feel that desire. But I do feel that women and periods – well, it's just a pain in the arse, it really is.

There was another thing I wanted to mention – I was hoping I'd do this in a sort of structured way, but I'm obviously not at all. I read an article about eight months ago, maybe a year ago, in *New Scientist*. It was about the menopause and Alzheimer's. Apparently, there are quite strong links between the menopause and Alzheimer's. I read that article and, this may now to some extent contradict other things I've said, but I was really close to tears. I was so upset by it and so afraid of what might happen to me. I feel I've had my fucking period my whole life and that's been a pain in the arse. I've had pregnancies I've not wanted, and I've had pregnancies that have ended in miscarriage. I didn't have children, but the whole thing around my period and fertility, I hate it. My father was a fertility expert so maybe there's a whole lot of psychoanalytical stuff going on there, who knows?

Then to discover that when you finally end the fucking thing, you might end up going mad and getting Alzheimer's because of it. I also felt that the tone of the article, which was written by a woman seemed somehow accepting of the idea that we have our menopause and become a bit hysterical and go a bit mad. Except it's worse than that. We literally go mad because we get Alzheimer's. Worse still, this is being scientifically proven. I just found myself thinking, 'We can't win.' What to do?

I don't know. I just wish my period would end, and I keep thinking, 'Is this really the menopause?' OK, I've had the night sweats and my periods have started becoming slightly erratic, so instead of being every twenty-seven days, it's now every twenty-one days. I get this from J because he's monitoring it, otherwise I wouldn't know.

But this is another thing – as you get older and you get closer to the ending, the bleeding gets closer together. I've had periods that are two and a half weeks apart. You just finish sticking tampons inside yourself and then you're starting all over again. I know it's not such a big deal, but on the other hand, it is, isn't it?

I remember the first time I put a tampon inside myself I found it a really distressing experience. I couldn't get it in you know, I was a teenager. The whole idea of poking something inside yourself. All of those memories and moments have stayed with me in such a powerful way that, for me, experiencing the moment it all ends is going to be so liberating and exciting.

Oh, and one last thing. I don't know how much detail to go into, but I have a healthy sex life and I think that when my periods end, it will get even better. This could be a complete fantasy on my part because it's not like my period gets in the way, but when I was younger it never used to bother me having sex while I was actually bleeding. As I've got older it has – I don't really want to have sex when I'm bleeding. So, you can imagine, now that my periods are every two and a half or three weeks, they frustrate me. 'It's my fucking period again!'

Sex is a massive part of it. For me it's one of the biggest parts of it. Here I am, aged fifty-one. I first had sex when I was relatively old, I think I was nineteen. Until very recently, sex was always a kind of anxiety, 'Will I get pregnant?' So, for my periods to end will be wonderful. It will finally mean that when I am having sex I will know, absolutely guaranteed, that there's no chance of getting pregnant.

I feel that with every sexual encounter I've had – and I was massively into sex (people say I shouldn't say promiscuous because it's a negative value judgement, so let's just say I've had a lot of sex) – I was always worrying, 'Am I going to get pregnant?' It's always there in the back of my head. So, I imagine that when my periods end, there will be a sense of abandon to me and to sex. I'll feel freer and so it's going to be even better. I'm really looking forward to that. I feel like the first time that I have sex when my periods have ended it's going to be fucking great – I just can't wait!

CHRISTINE

I feel that women are given a raw deal when you can feel so well on HRT.

I feel women are very underrepresented with HRT as they get older. I don't know whether this is because GPs are very aware of the cost of Hormone Replacement Therapy or HRT, but it does particularly annoy me. We give free contraception – which is basically a weaker version of HRT – to young girls from an early age. I realise it's for a good reason, and I used to work in Family Planning so, I mean, it is important. I just feel GPs – particularly female GPs and the young female ones – are not as keen to prescribe HRT. The older GPs tend to be a little bit more sympathetic.

I just think older women get a raw deal, but I've been taking it since I was forty-six which is quite young, but this was round about the time HRT had been sort of discovered, for want of a better word. I had a perimenopausal blood test and I was perimenopausal, not actually menopausal. A lot of people say that's a better time to start taking it, before you're actually into the symptoms.

I was going back into nursing – I'd been out of it and I decided to do a B. Tech and go back into nursing. The girls I was with were of a similar age and we knew that HRT was very current. One or two of us did decide to go and have a blood test – terrible isn't it! I was perimenopausal. My periods were still quite regular, but I was told that my oestrogen was lower than it should be. I started to take HRT and began to feel better, much more energetic. I'm going back now though; I mean I'm eighty next year. I was forty-six then, so it's been a long time.

I've had both my bunions done and this was probably about twenty years ago, and I had to come off the HRT for that. I don't think they'd take you off it now, but they did then. I came off for three months, and I really noticed. First thing I noticed was aching joints. I was about sixty. I honestly feel HRT has helped my joints, and just generally I feel well with it.

I've had no menopausal symptoms *at all*. When I became – what age – probably about sixty, they halved the amount of oestrogen which I accepted. It wasn't a dramatic change. I don't think I got any particular symptoms.

The only thing I notice now is that I can't remember as well, but I don't think that's HRT – I think it's more my age. My mum had Alzheimer's, so it's probably a weakness in the family.

Since I started taking HRT and, as I said, I'm still taking it now, the pros and cons have altered throughout the years. At first, they really plugged the fact that it was beneficial for the cardio-vascular system and then there was a phase about ten years ago when they said that it increased the risk of problems – I don't know. But they're slowly changing their minds again. They think that it helps the HDL cholesterol, the high-density lipoprotein cholesterol. I think it's the HDL – it's the good one anyway (because there's good and bad cholesterol).

I don't know what else I can say apart from, as I said earlier, I feel that women are given a raw deal when you can feel so *well* on HRT. I was told that if you actually went to the doctor now and were given HRT because you'd started the menopause, they would only probably consider for five years. I mean, I don't know because I don't deal with anybody who has HRT.

When I went for a repeat prescription for my HRT to a young female doctor – she was quite new – she said she didn't want to take responsibility for giving someone of my age HRT, and said I'd have to see the senior partner. I have oestrogen and progesterone tablets because I still have a womb. Of course, if you have a hysterectomy and have your uterus removed you wouldn't have both, just oestrogen. They didn't offer the patch when I went on it.

My main thing is, I feel that GPs don't give older women HRT. I also think it's unfair when they give young girls the pill. I mean I realise they're giving them it for a reason, and I do go along with that because, as I say, it was part of my job. But they're probably doing that, so they don't have to support unmarried mums. You know, I think it might be done for a social reason whereas with older women all they do is pay – the GP pays the bill. It's all down to money.

JOANNA WRITES

Rewilding the menopause

A couple of years ago at a weekend long retreat in Dartmoor I learned how to make fire from sticks, and baskets from switches of hazel. Our teacher, a buckskin-clad woman called Lynx, was visiting from the American West where she lives in a yurt and practises ancestral skills. One night she asked us to place ourselves around the campfire in age order. At fifty-one, I was the oldest woman in the group.

'As elders,' Lynx said addressing me and a sixty-something Frenchman called Bernard, 'what would you like to pass on to the younger generation?'

Bernard said some very funny and wise things.

It was my turn.

'Menopause,' I blurted, 'is wonderful!' The fire popped and sparks flew. 'It's not something to be afraid of; it's a trip.' These words had come from somewhere very deep and took me by surprise. Despite being in the thick of menopause, I had not spoken about it to anyone.

The next morning at breakfast several young women approached to say they'd never heard anything positive about menopause. They were hungry for more. I knew when I went on this retreat that I would be getting closer to the Earth, I would be camping and foraging for food, but I hadn't expected that in doing so I would get closer to my body.

It took being out in the wild to come to the shocking realisation that the thing preventing me from opening up about menopause was shame. I am embarrassed at losing my fertility, at seeing my looks fade, at getting old. In our youth-obsessed, consumer culture where surface beauty is valued along with our ability to make babies and stay 'hot', where would I find my currency as a middle-aged woman?

The word 'menopause' comes from the Greek *meno* for 'moon' – also the root for 'month' – and 'pause' meaning to 'halt'. Technically menopause is our last menstrual cycle. The correct term for the stretch of time from perimenopause until a year after our final period is the 'climacteric', which stems from the Greek word for 'ladder' and is also where we get 'climax'. Looking at menopause as a dramatic event, 'climax' fits nicely.

For centuries menopause was understood to be a deficiency disease. Our loss of oestrogen was not considered a normal physiological function of aging, but an illness. In Victorian times, the 'insanity' brought on by menopause was treated with poisonous purges of lead and mercury, sedation and incarceration in an asylum. It was also recommended that women's ovaries – their 'organs of crisis' – be removed. This, however, often proved lethal. In looking at its history, you begin to form a picture of menopause as a deadly business. Put bluntly, many women have died in the never-ending search for a 'cure' for its symptoms. When we weren't being physically dismembered or drugged, Freudians like Helene Deutsch, founder of the Vienna Psychoanalytic Institute, dissected our psyches. In her 1945 opus, *The Psychology of Women*, she argues that a woman's mental health was inseparable from her desire to be a mother and that women who embraced the end of their fertile years were 'deviant, unfeminine, and shameful'.

Women have always been victims of what Susan Sontag called the 'double standard of ageing'. Men can seamlessly graduate from boy to man but for women there is no equivalent: 'The single standard of beauty for women dictates that they must go on having clear skin. Every wrinkle, every line, every grey hair, is a defeat . . . even the passage from girlhood to early womanhood is experienced by many women as their downfall, for all women are trained to want to continue looking like girls.'

It was the swinging sixties that ushered in the way for middle-aged women to remain girl-like. This came in the form of physician Robert A. Wilson's 1966 bestseller *Feminine Forever*. In it he promised that his prescribed oestrogen therapy (ERT) would allow us to retain our 'straight-backed posture, supple breast contours, taut, smooth skin on face and neck, firm muscle tone, and that particular vigour and grace typical of a healthy female. At fifty, such women still look attractive in tennis shorts or sleeveless dresses.' On the other hand, if we failed to take these prescribed hormones 'from puberty to the grave' we became 'flabby', 'shrunken', 'dull-minded', 'desexed' 'castrates' who risked 'alcoholism, drug addiction, divorce and broken homes.' It gets worse: 'After menopause . . . the breast begins to shrivel and sag . . . Often the skin of the breast coarsens and is covered with scales.'

Scales! Wilson wasn't looking to alleviate menopause; he was looking to eradicate it lest we become monsters.

Here he is in predator mode: 'Roving about at a party, a footloose male might scan his surroundings at floor level, searching for a pair of trim legs . . . He assesses her face . . . her hands, teeth and throat.' Reading Wilson's book today is shocking. His abhorrence of our bodies is visceral and his distaste for the ageing process in women is violent, even sadistic. I could barely finish it.

Wilson's aggressive promotion of oestrogen was as materialistic as it was misogynistic: the writing of *Feminine Forever* and his book tours were funded by the companies who were manufacturing oestrogen and looking for a market. He received millions of dollars from pharmaceutical giant Wyeth, among others. In its first seven months, *Feminine Forever* sold 100,000 copies. Bafflingly, this book-length advertisement is still popular. 'A must-read for all women over 45!' ends one Amazon review from 2013.

Conjugated equine oestrogen (CEE), the hormone Wilson advocated was – and still is – manufactured from the urine of pregnant mares. If you're prescribed HRT today in the US or the UK, the chances are it will be Premarin (short for 'pregnant mares' urine'). And if you're squeamish, do not read to the end of this paragraph. The urine needed for ERT and HRT will have been extracted from mares held captive in horse farms in China, western Canada or the US. These creatures are tied up and kept pregnant, with catheters permanently strapped to their urethras. After about twelve years, they 'wear out' and are slaughtered. Their foals are sold for meat. But none of this will be discussed during your visit to the doctor. It's just another cog in the Big Pharma machine. And the chances are you won't be told about bio-identical hormones made from yam and soy, but these are beginning to get backing from the medical establishment.

'Almost any tranquiliser might calm her down, but at her age oestrogen might be what she really needs,' claimed an ad for Wyeth in the Journal of the American Medical Association in 1975 – the height of ERT uptake. Despite advertisements like this, and Wilson's contemptible proselytising, many feminists embraced oestrogen therapy. It would, they believed, release them from the trap of biological destiny. It wasn't so long ago that 'natural' processes such as childbirth often killed us, so the quest to be free from the diktats of our bodies is understandable.

However, the HRT honeymoon was not to last. By the mid-seventies, several drug companies in the US had been selling dangerous and untested products, such as the intrauterine contraceptive device known as the Dalkon Shield which killed thirty-six women and hospitalized a further 7,900. Then there was DES (Diethylstilbestrol), prescribed to prevent miscarriages and to alleviate the symptoms of menopause. The only problem was it had no positive effect on those conditions. It did, however, cause vaginal, cervical and breast cancer, auto-immune diseases and a whole host of abnormalities in many girls whose mothers had taken the drug. Those who were on the fence about hormone therapy started to rethink the trustworthiness of Big Pharma.

The health campaigner and journalist Sandra Coney wrote in her 1991 *The Menopause Industry*, 'Mid-life women have actually had no say in the services being provided for them. The "choices" available to them have been largely selected by commercial interests who have products and services to sell . . . The industry that has grown up around the provision of choices to mid-life women is primarily controlled by men.' Looked at like this, why would we want to trust the very men who are out to make money from our symptoms?

I am writing this from the frontline of menopause: hot flushes, night sweats, forgetfulness, and truly bizarre dreams overwhelm me both regularly and randomly, like guerrilla attacks. Maybe it's my love of stories, of always wanting to follow leads, but I cannot help but read these as part of a narrative – encouraged perhaps by the idea that I am indeed at a climax in this narrative.

If I silence this metamorphosis, this strange falling away of my old self, then how will I be able to mourn its loss and welcome its renewal? All of my symptoms feel wild, unprocessed and extreme – like the weather, like an avalanche or a tidal wave. At any moment, I have no idea what is about to hit. Are we not wired for this any longer? If we could accept the wild in us, would this not help us face the parts of ourselves that ebb and flow out of our control? Perhaps our inner wilderness, despite its sometimes inhospitable landscape, is really the last remnant of ourselves from a time when we, and everything around us, were wild. Could our domestication be preventing us from walking this landscape?

The popular advice coming at me on the subject of menopause made me angry. Jenni Murray's chirpy book, *Is it me or is it hot in here?* from 2001 gets very excited by the shiny hair and line-free skin enabled by HRT, without properly delving into the dangers: 'It will be a few years yet before we really know the benefits or otherwise of taking Hormone Replacement Therapy. Until then, we're all just guinea pigs in what may prove to be the greatest or the worst thing for women's health.' This understatement sadly came back to haunt Murray when she was diagnosed with breast cancer linked, she believes, to her HRT. She later wrote a piece in the *Telegraph* in which she confesses: 'So, if I had known then what I know now, would I have taken it? The answer is no. I now know that the menopause is a pain, but it doesn't last forever. Breast cancer, on the other hand, even if you survive it and I'm now in my tenth year, never leaves you.'

Too many of the conversations I hear around me focus on what brand of mare's urine I should be smearing on my thighs, or what diet I need to be on to stay sexy, despite my age. This is not what I am looking for. I want to interpret the symptoms, understand them, not eradicate them.

Because there is so little in the mainstream about reframing our attitudes towards women and ageing, I turned to anthropologists Faye Ginsburg and Rayna Rapp who tell us that, 'Menopause can never be understood apart from other social circumstances – marriage status, fertility history, access to property – through which women's power and experiences are constructed.' They go on, 'our own culture's conflation of . . . the loss of biological fertility with a reduction in status, is challenged by the fact that in many other societies post-menopausal women may adopt and foster children and have new authority over kin, especially daughters and daughters-in-law.' Finally! Here was a view of menopause that placed it in a wider context as a fluid and natural physiological process with myriad cultural, historical and personal interpretations, rather than as a monolithic obstacle to be drugged out of existence. Organisations like the Red School or Hands Inc. are working more in this vein.

Among some of the women I have spoken to, this social perspective is crucial. Friends who were sent into a premature menopause due to chemotherapy had to deal with the symptoms of their illness, the loss of parts of their bodies, the challenge of chemo itself and the even more profound distress of facing their mortality. Some feel 'aggrieved' at having menopause 'forced on them' and not being able to 'experience it naturally', which will inevitably mark their menopause specifically for them. Among those who wanted children but didn't manage to have any, menopause represents an acute and very private pain all of its own.

One friend who became suicidal turned to HRT, which she feels 'saved' her. Another found intercourse too painful and claims HRT brought the joy back into her sex life. I am not demonising anyone for choosing HRT, but I do wonder whether we would find it easier to bear our symptoms if society valued us for our accrued wisdom rather than our pert breasts.

Most of us at some point in our lives have struggled to accept our bodies. I don't need to list the statistics – we all know girls and women with eating disorders, who are full of self-hatred, who desire to be other than what they are. Menopause is no exception.

In order for us to begin to understand it, it might help to look into why menopause exists. The only other female mammals to live beyond their reproductive years are pilot whales and killer whales (orcas). The theory behind this is called the Grandmother Hypothesis.

Almost uniquely, orcas live in multi-generational pods: their offspring don't leave to set up their own family units but stay together as a tribe. If female killer whales were to carry on reproducing until death, their focus would be shifted away from the generations of existing offspring – but this doesn't explain the theory fully. It took Darren Croft and Ken Balcomb, scientists at Exeter University, to pin it down. Since the 1970s they have been studying killer whales in the Pacific Northwest, and the answer they have come up with is: salmon. These unpredictable fish make up 97 per cent of an orca's diet. 'They're not distributed equally in space,' says Croft. 'There are hotspots that differ with season, year, tide.' Because of their accumulated wealth of knowledge, the older females are more skilled at finding food when stocks are scarce or particularly unpredictable. 'Adult females are more likely to lead a group than adult males, and older post-menopausal females (who make up a fifth of the pod) are more likely to lead than younger ones. This bias was especially obvious in seasons when salmon stocks were low.'

A reliance on older women with their stores of accrued wisdom was a common thread in hunter–gatherer societies, which is perhaps what Lynx was keying us into around that campfire. Today however, adult women are encouraged to be silicon replicas of their younger selves. The knowledge we gain as we age is getting lost or being devalued and yet, as I saw in Dartmoor, the hunger for it is there.

But there is something else going on here, to do with the colonisation of the female body. Undoing my domestication and calling back something wild are the messages that keep coming at me from my hot flushes, night sweats and outlandish dreams. Germaine Greer, in her visionary 1990 book *The Change*, posits that menopause is a time to slow down, take stock and feel liberated from one's sexual objectification as well as from one's sexual desires. She advocates reclaiming the idea of the witch, the wise woman, the elder. And with our 'scaly breasts', why not? For me this is another opportunity in the narrative of menopause: Could we rewrite our stories and turn them into something more open-ended? Should we be exploring the unfamiliar plot lines, the places in ourselves we haven't been to? If we're lucky, our partners will come with us on the journey. Without dismissing those women for whom HRT is the difference between surviving menopause and not, I do wonder if a reframing of our worth as humans might help us cope where hormones can't. Recent studies in Europe and North America suggest a correlation between the severity of a woman's menopausal symptoms and her sense of being valued.

Despite all the good that the pharmaceutical industry has given us – the life-saving drugs, the cures for childhood diseases – it is fair to say that Big Pharma can be rapacious and reckless. I do not want the changes going on inside me to be silenced with drugs. I want to learn this new language coming at me deep from inside my body. At the moment, I have gleaned a few words, and so far they are telling me this: stop, be quiet, and listen, only then will you understand.

HILARY

New, 2007

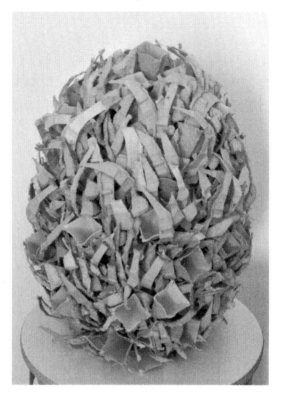

Shown at the *Spitz gallery in 2007*, this sculpture is formed from pieces cut from egg boxes, which are reassembled to form an egg shape. The transformation, not only from the function of the original material but also to a new more beautiful object, suggests a bud of new growth.

JULIE

Although I used to think I'd be so bloody relieved when I stopped having periods, I think I will miss it because it's been such a big part of my life since I was fifteen years old, and I think I will miss it.

I am currently perimenopausal so, from what I understand, I am not in menopause yet but I'm going through the stages that lead up to the menopause. There are certain changes going on in my body physically, mentally and emotionally. My understanding is that I'm getting ready for *the change*.

I'm Bengali, born and brought up in the east end of London. I'm working class, brought up in council housing, so I'm from a particular demographic, I would say. I went to University – well, it was a polytechnic but became a University by the time I left. I straddle different social classes. I'm not working class like my parents were, but I don't own my own house. Being a woman from an ethnic minority growing up in London, I think, defines me culturally.

I'm fifty years old. My mum, from what I remember, had quite an early menopause. It was quite tumultuous. She'd get really moody and all sorts of things, so I'm not sure when she actually went through it, but I remember us being young. We never had conversations about the menopause or women's health generally. These sorts of things were never really discussed in my family. We just got on with it when we had to do stuff and had to work it out for ourselves.

There's probably a word in Bengali for Menopause, but I don't know it. I think there must be because it's such a big deal culturally in South-east Asia – there are certain things you can't do if you're on your period. Like for Hindu women they can't go to the temple, so the fact that someone's past their fertility would be significant and noticeable. It's quite a ritualised culture, so although there might not be conversations about it, it would be obvious because of the way you interact in your community as to whether you were fertile or not. Women who are married wear red, so after a certain period if you're not active like that you're not seen in the same way – there's a different value given to those women, they're usually seen as widows. It's the same in the West. Women who are fertile are valued in a particular way compared to women who are not fertile. But, yes, in the Bangladeshi community there are clear indications and signs that you're not fertile anymore. I just don't know enough about if there is a word for it because I can only speak a dialect of Bengali and I don't read and write in it and I've never studied it, so I don't really know.

The physical effects on the body are the things that I've noticed most – the changes in body temperature when I sleep at night. Also, I get tired, I get irritable, and it has affected my libido – I don't really want sex as much as I did before. Emotionally and mentally I find things more challenging definitely, especially if I'm going through a difficulty. I tend to be more upset, weepy, emotional or depressed. I feel like I go beyond the appropriate response – it becomes much more intensified and my reaction is much more irrational.

I've learnt that physical activity and exercise really do help me to balance that out. I find going swimming regularly is really useful. It's not just the physical for me – it's also the mental space for me to be able to unclutter things in my head. Also, there's something about doing something in the water – just swimming up and down really calms me down and makes me feel connected in my body and mind in a way that's really more harmonious which is really good – it helps with my mood.

I do yoga too which I also find really useful. I only do it once a week because I haven't got much time – I'd like to do it more. The practice is about breathing – it's about doing the poses but also doing exercises that make us much more present in our bodies. I think this helps a lot because there's a lot of disconnection between ourselves and our bodies – and that's not just for women who are menopausal. I think a lot of people don't feel very connected to their physical body most of the time – they're in their heads. I think it would help to be much more connected physically because we'd be more aware of our responses – how a situation might affect us physically, and we'd be a bit more present.

Definitely there is a strong link with ageing for me. I feel I am an older woman now – because I'm approaching menopause and don't feel youthful in the way I used to. I don't have that kind of energy. I don't feel the same sort of inclinations as well, so there's been a shift in the way that I think about life, my values, my attitudes. In the past I would've been much more about acquiring experiences, doing new things, chasing after ... whatever. Now I'm quite happy just to let things happen. If I'm happy doing whatever, I'm quite happy just to do it. I'm not so eager to acquire things or experiences.

I'm much more settled in myself, so I don't feel the need to be aspirational in that sense. That drive isn't there – it might be the fact that I am older, or it might be the fact that I've decided that there are different things that are important to me. But I think it is related to being older, to be honest, and wanting different things out of life. Knowing that I'm approaching a part of my life that will be different to what it was before, and that awareness affects me.

I've never had children and I've never wanted to have children. I don't feel sad about it, I don't regret it, I don't feel the need to justify my life by having children, but there *is* a part of me that thinks, 'Oh, what would it have been like to be a mum?' It's a part of being a woman and female that I haven't experienced, so there's always that question mark. It's OK that I have that though.

There have been many effects on my cognition. I was never great at remembering things anyway, but now I tend to get even more muddled, more confused, especially if I'm juggling things. I find that I miss things out a lot, so there has been an effect on my ability to think and reason and try and work things out. I can still do all the things I want to do, that's important.

My cousin was put on HRT when she had her uterus removed, and she's felt fine on it. She did want to have children, so it was a huge blow to her that she couldn't. HRT has helped her maintain a sense of being herself, and that's really important to her. She hasn't felt that she's lost anything. Yes, she's lost her uterus, but she hasn't lost who she is – she's still got the energy, she's still got a sense of who she used to be and none of that has gone away, so I think HRT can be really positive for people. I know friends and aunties who've been on HRT and I don't really know anyone whose had negative experiences of it but, because people don't talk about it very much it's not really something I'd necessarily know. Often people don't like to talk about their problems because they think it's boring or irrelevant or they feel inadequate or like they're failing in some way.

I don't have a position on HRT. I don't know how I'm going to experience the menopause and whether I'll need it or not. At the moment it seems like it's OK, but I might get to a point where I'm not coping and I'll probably ask for support or help from my GP and I don't know what they'll offer me, so I'll have to deal with that if that time comes.

I wouldn't say I identify as middle-aged. I feel I'm an *older* woman, but I don't feel middle-aged. I don't know if I even went through middle-age. I feel that I was young and now I'm older, so I'm not sure what middle-age is. It seems to be a vague definition of age. For me, anything like thirty and under is young, anything sort of fifty plus is older – I don't feel middle-aged, but maybe I am. I just know I'm not young anymore. Back in the day, I would have been dead by now. The goal posts change as we get older. When I was young, I remember thirty seeming really old and I remember thinking, 'I hope I'm dead by then,' sort of thing! Now, for me, old is like ninety. I know people that age who are still active or not active, and they're still knocking about and getting things done. So, you know, it's not inconceivable that people survive a long time.

So, I probably am middle-aged, but I don't feel it. I kind of think of middle-aged people as a bit younger still. In Tower Hamlets you get special discounts and things when you're fifty, so it's *seen* as old. If you go to the gym or something, you'll get a discount, cheaper rates if you're fifty and use the facilities – there's the 'Young at Heart' thing for people of fifty plus. So, it's different for different people.

I think I'm going to be working for a long time to come. I don't think I'm going to be stopping working soon, even though people retire at sixty-five, or is it older now? It'll go up – it keeps going up. I'm not in a position to retire, so I'll have to keep working. As long as I'm able to be, I think I'll be active.

When I was growing up, I was always clear about what I wanted to do in life – as I get older, I'm less clear and less sure about the things I want and what I'm doing. I still feel quite sure of who I am, though, and I know the things I don't want, let's say, even if I don't know what I do want. This is quite important – I know what I won't accept.

I am actually upset – a part of me is upset – that I will be going through the menopause. Although I used to think I'd be so bloody relieved when I stopped having periods, I think I will miss it because it's been such a big part of my life since I was fifteen years old, and I think I will miss it. I thought I'd be really relieved not to have a single period ever again, but I'm thinking, 'Maybe I will miss it', for whatever reason. So, that's something that's surprised me.

MARCELLE

I think we need to get it out in the open and for women to feel it's not something to be dreaded, but something to be curious about really, and see ...

An interesting aspect which I have been reflecting on is that when you are menopausal it means that you will lose your sexual attraction to the world in general, or that is the assumption. You start to smell differently, in that you don't smell anymore as a possible biological woman on heat because, you know, all that disappears.

You become like a nobody. You're not seen, and you have no value in a way. Yes, I guess for a lot of women you have no value in the game of – well, sexual games, power games, of being counted.

As for men, they will maybe not even reflect on this or acknowledge it, but I think subconsciously it is definitely there. I think a lot of men would not like the idea that they, in their forties or even in their early fifties, would make love to a menopausal woman or a woman who has gone through it.

It's not that they want children, but it's the *old hag* association, which is quite curious as, contrary to that, in these present times, women look a lot younger for a lot longer. Women far into their sixties or even in their seventies might be sexually attractive, or at least look like they're interested. They dress well, they have fewer worries, they will maybe have more money because they've had kids who have grown up, or whatever, and they are more confident because they have made their careers and found out, more or less, who they are. All these kinds of things make them more attractive and, yet, the fact is that they are sexually on the trash heap, on the slag heap – they just don't really count anymore.

I think it is a very primitive kind of feeling, so a lot of people will be quite secretive about the fact that they have a menopause.

You know, you can have hot flushes, you can also become quite forgetful. I've always been half forgetful, though I'm sure it became worse with my menopause. But it's almost like you have to excuse yourself, 'Oh, I'm *sorry* I have the hot flushes, I'm *sorry* I'm forgetful, it must be my menopausal kind of mind.' This excusing is as if, well, you're not ill though you're not as vigorous and perfect as before, whether you were perfect then or not.

I was on HRT for fifteen years – it was a very long time, because I had an early menopause in my early forties. At the time there was *no-one* who could give me answers because no-one talked about it. My mother said, 'I can't remember.' I asked other people of her age and they said they couldn't remember. It was definitely something you'd have to suffer in silence or, if it was really bad, just go to the doctor and get some pills.

There is no sense of a kind of celebration or entering a different stage in life altogether. It is a signpost, you know, at whatever time in your life it happens. It is also a *freedom* – you can make everlasting love without ever having to take any pills. You don't have to worry about anything like that, because you can't get pregnant anymore.

But also, and I think more importantly, you have arrived at a stage in your life in which you are *returning home* to yourself as a person. It is the beginning of the coming home to yourself. This is not in an idealistic, 'Oh god, I'm so wise and smart and I've seen it all and done it all,' but there is a kind of completeness about you because that uncertainty of getting confirmation from other people that you are acceptable or that you are somebody (from men often or from society) has become irrelevant. It's not that men have no voice, but you don't need to have that affirmation from them to feel complete. And, in a way, because you won't get it, as you're not fertile anymore, it sets you free to say, 'Ok, I'm going to function in a different way now. I don't need to … how to say it … *manipulate* anything to get a share in the power'. The power is yours now, and it's not about having power over someone, but just that you are strong in yourself.

It's not really, you know, a time when you're going to have a complete change of career. You are where your feet are leading you, that kind of thing. Some things you're interested in might develop into a career, but you're not saying, 'Oh yes, now I'm fifty I really want to be an air stewardess of something, or a fire fighter, or whatever', like when you're sixteen or eighteen.

I think it is a very *liberating* thing and I regret that it is rarely, in our western society, celebrated as a transition. It's like your period which, I think too, is also rarely celebrated in this society.

As you become a woman it is always, 'Oh, it's their emotions or it is smelly.' When I first heard the expression *the curse* in the English language, I thought it was a very odd word for it – it's not like that in Dutch. In Dutch the word is *ongesteld* which means that you're ill – or, more accurately, you're not feeling well. It's not a curse, first of all. It is the *essence* of life, but really using the word curse sort of explains a negative attitude about menstruation. I think that the menopause also has that negative attitude instead of it being a natural kind of progression.

You're going into the next stage of life before old age and illness starts. It is sequential, and I think it is quite a *flowering* of life. I see a lot of women who are actually flowering after the menopause or with the menopause because they are free of a lot of things and yet it is still something that, in general, women don't want other women to know, or other men to know. It is slightly like there is something *off* about you, like the food you buy that is out of date though still perfectly edible, it's out of date therefore no good. I have food in the fridge that can be two or three weeks out of date, but often it's alright and I can eat it.

Obviously, physically there are women who have an absolutely terrible time, really terrible. I have no experience of that, but I know people who have and, of course, for them the menopause is definitely a *curse-like* situation, and it can last a long time.

I went for HRT basically because nobody could give me any answers, I was totally confused. I was quite moody and all that in my head. I thought that it must be the menopause, so I got a blood test and it said yes, confirmed it. I then said, 'Can you tell me a bit about it?', and they said, 'No, just take HRT.' This was at the Family Planning Clinic, and they really wanted me to shut-up, take the hormones and just behave, that was it.

I did, basically, because I was so confused and there was nobody I could ask and get a decent answer from. My parents didn't answer anything like that, older women who had been through their menopause said they couldn't remember and because my menopause started quite early I couldn't ask people of my age. I couldn't get much information – this was before the time of the internet, more or less. Books weren't really any help – this was in the eighties, maybe eighty-five or eighty-nine, I can't remember exactly.

I took HRT – I didn't have a period with it – and everything went back to being my normal self, whatever that was. So, it didn't become an issue to enquire about menopause and all that. I didn't pay much attention to it to be honest. Then, at some point I thought, 'OK, I can take HRT till I die, but maybe this is enough, I don't want to keep taking hormone pills,' so I thought, 'Why don't I just stop it and see how it goes?', and I did.

I was sixty when I stopped the HRT. I don't know if it was connected to HRT or to the lifeforce rearing its head one more time before old age started, but I had a roaring libido for about seven years. I had several affairs with old flames etc, partly to correct the past which, of course, is not possible.

Creatively, in my work as an artist, it was also a great time.

I did then have hot flushes, but not terrible. It was quite funny, you know. You'd go into a shop and because of the temperature change from the street to the shop you'd go *whoosh* and just walk straight out of the shop again. I have seen other women do it. You just burst out into a flush and say, 'Right, out you go!'. I didn't have terrible night sweats, so maybe by that time I had it out of my system. I didn't have violent periods either – I'm not sure that is disconnected, to be honest.

I think that lasted maybe a year, maybe a year and a half or something. Afterwards I had a slight regret, in a way, that I had missed out on some sort of *sharing* the kind of ritual of transformation. It was like a *nothing*, same as my periods had been.

When I got my period, nobody talked about it. My mother got me some sanitary towels and gave me a book about sexuality that I didn't understand – it was a medical kind of book. It was like a non-event while it is a *big* event, a *big* change in your life both physically and for your inner life. I'm not saying that you have to have sort of baby shower ideas for it, but I think it would be nice when it happens, to get a group of friends together, male and female, and mark it. To say, 'Hey, listen, something is happening to me – there's a difference in my life, and an irreversible difference.'

I feel, all together, that the whole notion of old age is still negatively viewed in our society, especially old age for women. For men, somehow, looking like some kind of dried prune or something is always interesting, but I think women have to look slim or if you're really old you have to look like Iris Apfel with her big glasses and all that. I feel that this whole idea of old age is not disconnected with the menopause.

Old age can have so many forms until you get ill of course – that's another kind of step. But I think old age is not just like being a babushka and giving wisdom to people, but progressively you enter a stage of greater privacy and freedom and, also, approachability. I find often, not that people seek me out, but loads of people talk to me all the time. There's a kind of relaxation because you're not a threat, you know, in a sexual way. People don't have to fear that if they say something or do something it will be misconstrued – all these kinds of things sort of fall away, and so people can have a greater kind of freedom in being themselves.

I find it very interesting that when I was in my twenties I thought that people that were older than me were just in a different world. We didn't talk to them, like we didn't talk to grandparents or anything, just kept secrets from them. They were just old!

So, I think the society has changed a lot and for the better in many, many ways and certainly for women – fantastic strides for women. I'm not saying we're there, but the fact that we have a lot of individual freedom I think is absolutely brilliant.

At the same time, there is still this very conservative trend that you have to tick the boxes all the time of being sort of slim, beautiful and sexy. And then you think, 'Yes, right, when I was slim, beautiful and sexy, I wanted people to like me for my mind.' I mean, you can't win! So, let's just drop the whole thing and just see how things go.

But I think it's more the *concept* of menopause which *really* should change collectively. I also think men should be involved, for them to understand what happens to women's bodies and to their whole being. You know, they are part of our world – we share the world together, so they should not be not excluded and just say, "I'm not going to talk to her, she's menopausal", or think you're moody and slamming a door because your menopausal or it's your period, when really you slam the door because you're pissed off that you forgot your umbrella or something and got wet. It's like, 'Go away, I'm just slamming the door because I've been stupid, or I'm annoyed, or something.'

I think we need to get it out in the open and for women to feel it's not something to be dreaded, but something to be *curious* about really, and see ...

It's a more reflective time that happens – not for everyone, obviously, but I think there is generally more reflection.

EDIE WRITES

A few words

I don't think I have anything to contribute.

My menopause was a total non-event.

I might have had a tiny hot flush once, maybe.

I feel that I have failed the sisterhood!

LAURA

My friend said that her specialist said to her, 'Only Ladies that lunch can cope with the menopause. If they have a job, they should take HRT', so she does.

I think it's confusing because it's hard to know what the menopause is and what it isn't. I only had my child thirteen years ago, so I think a lot of things started around then and perhaps kind of continued. Things like not sleeping, for example, has been an issue since pregnancy really. But I think it's more persistent now. It's really, really hard not sleeping, because you never feel like you'll get total oblivion. Not to have a single night without that oblivion does wreak havoc with your mental state, I think. You're always fighting tiredness. Luckily, I've got the kind of job where you can sort of disappear for a day, as in I can work from home. If I had to be present and visible on a daily basis

I think it would be really, really difficult at the moment, but I can have a day when I can work on the computer for a few hours and then, if I have to, I can go and slump in a heap for a bit and then re-surface on line. Yes, so that's really hard.

Also, anxiety, I guess, really is a feature. I know I've spoken to friends who've said the same thing. One of my friends, she said, 'It's come from nowhere', but I know what it's like to feel anxious having had Post Natal Depression, though that felt different. I think it's more of a kind of low-lying dread feeling and you don't really know what that's about – an existential feeling. Maybe it's combined with being tired. I sometimes feel like I'm kind of looking in on my life and not really participating in it, just going through the motions a bit. But my job is quite convenient in that it can be all consuming. Although I've said that I don't have to be visible, it's the kind of job you could do for ten hours, and you could do at the weekend and still not feel like you're done. So, although it's tiring, it's convenient because I can just kind of lose myself in it.

When I'm not working, I can feel a bit spaced out and a bit kind of empty, I guess, but that could be due to ageing and thinking all my milestones have passed. Seeing your life post-fifty is very different to pre-fifty, I think. Whether that's a symptom of the menopause I don't know. But, yes, I find that upsetting, just kind of not feeling I'm in my life. So, even at Christmas I felt like that – just going through the motions and, actually, just wanting everyone gone, just really wanting to be alone a lot – people are draining. We were visiting the in-laws in their new house and we'd had days of socialising. When we came back I just said, 'I'm going to bed. It's half past seven. I cannot cope with people anymore.' So, yes, I just find lots of company very draining.

I feel over-stimulated by things sometimes as well, and highly irritated – more irritated than before perhaps. So sometimes I'm deep breathing while listening to R (my daughter) and feeling, 'I'm so irritated at the moment, I just want to scream'. I know that I'm being unreasonable and that she's just venting, so I just kind of give the impression that I'm listening but actually inside I'm about to boil over – I just want her to go away.

I guess a lot of people go through the menopause with their children grown-up, you know, a very different stage. But I see it as a plus having a sort of youngish child still because it kind of keeps me young mentally as well and I have to focus on the here and now, put her first and all those things. I don't feel like I'm old or middle-aged in my attitudes. I know about the latest music, the latest street language and all that kind of thing, so I think having a younger child in some ways is a good thing when you're going through this.

In terms of the physiological I have more aches and pains I suppose, stiffness. I don't miss having periods – I'm not bothered about that. I guess for some women there's some mourning involved in that reduced fertility, but I'm not really worried about that.

I actually feel like having a big change. It would be nice to say, 'Right, draw a line under that, let's have a big change. Let's move house or start doing some of the things

I like doing.' But, because of the stage we're at with R being at school and being very much stuck into our jobs, that it isn't possible, but it would feel like the natural thing to do right now – to do something a bit radical. Yes, a new era kind of feeling – that would be quite nice. But instead, I just feel a bit like I'm going through the motions.

Waking up in the middle of the night it's kind of, 'What's this all about?' It's never a good thing to do, is it, waking at three in the morning? It's probably not possible to be cheerful. I guess that intensifies it doesn't it, wandering about the house at that hour? You can think, 'Let's see. If I go back to sleep again, I'll get five hours sleep, so that should be enough to crawl through the day. If I'm lucky I might just scrape six. It's OK, I can have an early night tomorrow, you know'. There's a lot of all that kind of thinking. And to be tired all the time is just not nice. When I do have a day when I've got energy it's amazing.

I went for a run for the first time in about thirty-five years on New Year's Day. I thought, 'Right, New Year's resolution, I'm going go for a run. Yes, I hate running, but I'm going to do it'. So, I kind of trotted to the park and then went on the machines and I felt great. It felt awful to start with, horrendous, but I felt good afterwards and thought, 'New me, this is what I'm going to do. I'm going to be the fittest I've been, I'm going to increase my bone density.' That Mariella Frostrup programme partly inspired me actually, the runners had the best bone density didn't they? I thought I can increase my bone density and banish the blues at the same time. So, you kind of know what's the answer, you know that'd be a good thing. I know if I did that it would really help, but it's finding the motivation, and I think when you feel flat it's quite difficult.

So, yes, you're just kind of stuck in the middle of it, aren't you? You just think, 'Is this just me? Is this menopause? Will it *ever* be different?'

I've got a colleague who's in his sixties, his wife's in her sixties as well. He said that their marriage nearly broke down when she had her menopause because, he used the phrase, 'She went into herself for about two years.' I don't know that he handled it very well. She didn't want him to come anywhere near her, she didn't want any physical contact or anything. I kind of recognise that – going into yourself just wanting to be on my own a lot, listening to K but not really hearing him, perhaps. He just seems so full of life and is so in the moment with his work and his business, and I can't really identify with that. Things that I want to do, you know, like travelling or just sort of seeing more natural beauty, music or just kind of those more nurturey type things, he's not in that space at all. He's very much in the business, making money, you know, the 'to do list' mentality, so we're kind of quite different. Yes, *very* different. I'm more existential, reflective and wanting things to nurture me. Hence, that's probably just why I just kind of work because work is quite comforting – it's comforting because you don't have to think about yourself so much.

But I guess there must be positives. You must hear lots of complaining about it. I don't want to paint too negative a picture about it but, as I said, it's hard to separate the wood from the trees,

I haven't had horrible hot flushes. I don't know when you're supposed to have those – whether you're supposed to have them once you're fully in it. I get hot in the night when I can't sleep and I'm throwing off the covers, though my mum says she still does that, so I'm assuming that kind of carries on which is really annoying, but I haven't had that during the day. It'd be quite nice not to have that – I don't know if everyone gets that or just a proportion of people.

So, physically I can't complain too much really, apart from the sort of fog. Have people said that to you? The brain fog. It kind of feels physical as well. Like at the moment I'm feeling it, like your head just feels heavy, stuffy. It's like you've got a cold, but you haven't, kind of jam-packed. It's a little bit spaced out, feeling light-headed. I had a dizzy moment the other day at the swimming pool when I got out. It was like 'Woah,' and I had to hold onto the wall – that was a bit weird. I was thinking, 'Oh god, what's that about?' but then I've read that dizziness can be a symptom and I can now identify with it.

It's also just feeling bit vague, so I'm always joking with people at work, saying, 'Just remind me because I'm quite forgetful at the moment about things.' So, I've been doing this brain app, this sort of brain training thing religiously, because I'm thinking, 'I've got to fight this.' Little things like that are kind of attempts on my part to keep things moving, keep things sharp. I think that's really important – to play the guitar, re-learn a language, that kind of thing. You have to fight it don't you? You can't just let it swamp you. I want to listen to more live music, see more films, keep my brain alive. I went to see an amazing film a couple of nights ago, so I'm just trying to do things a bit differently. That was good, anything like that, I think, that just takes me out of my head – a little bit different, a little bit unpredictable is good. I'm very much of the view that you have to fight things.

I don't take anything. I'm not taking any supplements. I tried green tea capsules for a while, but then there's some bloke in America who had to have a liver transplant. I thought, 'Bloody Hell'. I was so annoyed because it was actually really making a difference, and I don't think it was a placebo because I'd taken things in the past and thought, 'Oh, that's a load of rubbish', but I was actually feeing quite different with the green tea capsules, until I heard about the bloody man with his liver transplant. It's just one man, but I thought I'd knock that one on the head. I thought maybe I should get my liver function tested because if it wasn't having any impact then I'd think it was a good thing actually, but hey.

I don't take HRT or anything just because I've got an increased risk of breast cancer. I probably wouldn't take it anyway even if I didn't just because of the bad press it's had recently, but I'm sure it's a really good thing for lots of people. My friend said that her specialist said to her, 'Only Ladies that lunch can cope with the menopause. If they have a job, they should take HRT', so she does.

But, you know, you shouldn't really have to take something to cope with something that every woman has to endure – there must be other ways.

JOSEPHINE WRITES

A selection of diary entries from 1964 and 1966

Josephine's dairies were left to her daughter. The following are extracts that Josephine's daughter thinks are very likely to have been connected to her mother's menopause. Josephine uses an intriguing code at times: X and Y. X seems to be a positive experience, and Y a negative one.

1964

Jan 16th: Depression seems deeply rooted

Jan 23rd: I feel l must have some occupational therapy to prevent me sinking too deeply into depression.

Jan 28th: Wrote to T ... I sank into the deepest depression yet – just a feeling of inadequacy, struck all of a heap by it and not wanting to live at all. Everything seemed down.

Jan 29th: Feeling a bit better because one can't feel at the bottom all the time.

18th Feb: Feeling wretchedly unhappy – all remote unfriendly. Lack of any self-confidence – perhaps these surroundings make me feel unworthy. And I was so looking forward to this week.

23rd Feb: Feel rather depressed …

2nd March: Feeling very depressed and miserable. I wonder if these black moods are anything to do with the glands. Providing I keep them to myself and 'dear diary' I suppose they won't do any harm. Went to Harley St to see Dr about foot, which he says is OK and also skin irritation – he says antihistamine given last August should be a help. He says the shedding is a sign of <u>life</u> not death, and I needn't worry. Felt a bit better.

5th March: Washed my hair, a handful came out – just like August and very depressing.

9th *March*: Felt some real contentment for the first time in weeks (because glimpse of X), how long will it last?

12th March: Am back in the blues again – a nightmare state of apprehension. However, the smallest lightening of the gloom raises my spirits to false euphoria very easily.

13th March: I felt a little better, but it takes only a sudden changing of X to Y to push me down again.

14th March: I still tremble with nerves but feel a tiny bit more optimistic.

16th *March:* Optimism beginning to set in.

18th March: Washed hair and was surprised to have any left to set.

20th March: All very pleasant and happy. X indeed.

16th April: V started school. I feel quite empty of life and vitality and even of hope. Angry silence – and I lie at the bottom of snake pit and wish some malignancy (organic I mean) would carry me away without all the scandal and publicity that suicide would cause.

19th April: Woke with a slight pain in front of ears … hoped it was not mumps.

21st April: I still have mock-mumps but feel well.

22nd April: Pain seems to have gone so that flap over.

23rd April: Felt very tired and went to bed at 7.30 with a sandwich.

9th May: (Row with L) so 'back in the pit again.'

10th May: Feeling a bit more X, but I sometimes wonder 'how long?'

28th July: I was streaming with sweat.

11th August: I feel very contented here waiting for the next anxiety to start. Head so much better.

22nd August: I feel quite contented with none of the usual angsts, but I still wake in the dead of night for an hour or two.

1966

26th January: Have been very depressed and feeling on the edge of tears for no reason at all, but the prospect of keeping these things in flower is very heart-lifting.

1st Feb: The Vit B seems to be improving me to the extent that no longer so depressed, yet I get the horrors still when dropping off to sleep and the mornings are hellish from 7.15 to 8am as we get up at 7.30am.

11 Feb: Went to Dr for last injection of Vit B12. I think it has helped with the depression and 'vibes' but don't know whether much will be done for the hair.

17 Feb: Washed hair early in day. Wasn't coming out as much but seems much thinner.

25th February: Felt low all day. A rather frightening glimpse of Y over a triviality but I suddenly took fright after it and felt wretched, but it was all forgotten later, and my spirits soared again.

12th April: Awoke feeling flayed, reconciliation took place and X returned to me, but remained exhausted and limp for the rest of the day.

PENNY

I think that's why so many women get so angry – there's no choice – it's just put upon you.

My menopause started at thirty-six. I'm a mum with two boys, lived in Bethnal Green all my life. I had two beautiful, beautiful boys and then was suddenly hit by this *horrible, horrible* thing that came from nowhere. I was thrown advice by everyone from, 'Pull your socks up and get on with it', to HRT, to reading books. People were throwing advice, but no-one was actually *helping* me – that maybe doesn't make sense, but ...

Well, I was bombarded with books and lotions and potions and I didn't want that – I wanted someone to know what it was like to be going through it, to know that I wasn't going mad and that I wasn't going to go to the doctor's and them call an ambulance and section me!

After twenty-five years of marriage I still love my husband and I still love my children. I wanted the children to have that stability to come home and know that mum was not going to be 'nice mummy' or 'bad mummy'. It really hit home one day when I forgot my son's school play – he came in and the tears were rolling down his face and it was, 'I hate you mummy.' I had totally forgotten about this school play, the play that I had sat and made the costume for and practised the lines for. And he said, 'I wish you'd go away, and the old mummy come back.' It was a see-saw of emotions – and very, very lonely though – a very, very lonely place.

You question who you are, and you grieve. I was 36. I have two beautiful boys that I love to pieces and, you know, I would have taken the stars out of the sky for them, but I grieve for that child that I might have had. Maybe there was that one chance that there was a little girl that I could have had, and that was taken away from me.

And suddenly I didn't feel worthy as a person, as a mother, as a wife. It was this constant struggle with fatigue and dark days. Your menopause is very night and day sometimes. The night's the bad day, the light's the rainbow. So, the brighter the colour the better the mood, sort of thing.

And I'm nearly 11 years in now – there's no answers as to where it's going to go, but I've learnt to live with it. I've learnt to live with the menopause, and, through the support group, I've been very privileged to meet some wonderful, wonderful people and to share experiences and know that

I'm not alone. It's not some secret club, it's going to happen to every single woman.

And, that's my menopause.

After a few minutes break a few further thoughts occurred to Penny:

Eleven years in there's still good days and there's still bad days – some days it's absolutely fine and some days it's absolutely *awful* and there's still answers that I want. When is it going to end? That little pain in my back, is it a menopause pain or is it another pain? I suppose one of the advantages of starting earlier is that, hopefully, by the time I reach fifty it'll all be over, and I've got a good many years of happiness in front of me.

But, you know, I'll always grieve for that child, maybe that little daughter that I never had. But then life's full of ifs and maybes isn't it, but I'll always grieve and always think it was unfair that it happened so early and that my choice was taken away.

I think that's why so many women get so angry – there's no choice – it's just put upon you. If it was a broken leg or, it sounds extreme, but even cancer then they can try to treat you. Apart from HRT what can they do for the menopause? I just hope that maybe as time goes on and medical advances happen, we can treat it and maybe even shorten it, or even completely eradicate it maybe somehow. I don't know.

And that *is* my menopause.

PAULINE

Land

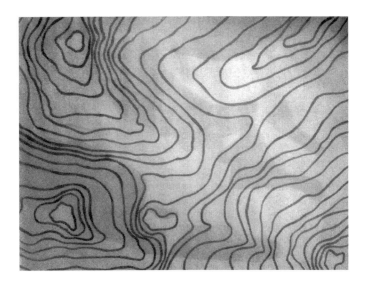

Flying high over a hot, dry desert land.

EMMA

*It's certainly a passage to be negotiated and I do think –
when will it end? Is there an ending? How do you know
when you're though it? It does end, doesn't it? Plenty of
people will have come out the other side.*

I was talking to someone this week about doing this,
another woman who's gone through the menopause. She
said, 'Well, actually, you know, menopause is technically
your last period. We've added all this other stuff to it and
now understand the menopause as a much wider process.'
That got me thinking about when my last period was. I'm
fifty-seven now and, of course, in a typically menopausal
way I can't remember. It was, I think, probably four or five
years ago and I remember, at the time, thinking that it was
related to something, that it was a significant day. Before
that, I suppose, I'd had nearly a year since having a period,

so I never quite knew when the ending was coming, because there'd been that year and then I had another one I thought 'I think this is the last knockings, I think this is going to be it'.

So, yes, I feel that I'm *very* much still in the menopause – I know that primarily by flushes. Thinking about doing this today, I was reflecting about how it's quite difficult maybe to separate things out because I have felt quite different in my fifties from my forties. What's actually hormonal, what's ageing, what's post-analysis? I finished psychoanalysis in my early fifties, so, you know, working out kind of what's what really. But I *definitely* have a sense of a 'change of life' in all sorts of ways, I suppose.

But just on the physical symptoms – the flushes still go on and I was thinking, actually, that I find them less invasive than periods. Finishing with periods was a quite good aspect of it for me. I was having very heavy periods every three weeks before I stopped and had to have medication because otherwise I just couldn't manage. I was flooding out and was also very drained by them, they were really very heavy. So, actually, to stop all that and replace it with flushes (which aren't very pleasant, but not as invasive or anxiety-provoking in a way as my periods got to be towards the end) is a good thing.

I think with the flushes, I get them a bit at night sometimes, but in my forties, I was a real insomniac in a very disturbing way – sometimes so much so that I wondered if I'd be able to work, and that sort of thing. I was very disturbed at night and couldn't get back to sleep and so, although I now never sleep through the night, I usually get back to sleep again. I'm not as disturbed as I was.

I think what I'm trying to do is put it in *context* that, yes, I'm very aware of physical things going on, but they're part of the trajectory which isn't any worse than it was before in different ways.

The *main* surprise and thing that I find most difficult is the sense of cognitive impairment. I wasn't ready for that and it's been *quite* a shock. I don't hear it talked about so much. I am hoping that some of it is a menopausal symptom, and I haven't got the early stages of Alzheimer's. I've noticed in so many different ways really, one is just memory. I used to have a very good memory and recall, and I'm noticing now a loss of that in all sorts of domains really. At work, when I met with people clinically, I used to be able to recall details of sessions for quite a long time afterwards whereas now if I don't write it down I can't remember it beyond the day. I have to write a lot of details down to remember what was going on, what I've done. Academically, I've almost got to the point where I don't see the point of reading papers because I can't remember them. I have the immediate hit of reading something and it makes sense and I suppose there may be one or two salient points which I hold on to, but if you ask me to say what the paper was about in any kind of depth I'd really struggle to remember it.

And then, just on a more day to day basis, I've noticed time feels very different. I used to have a sort of sense of continuity about what I did last week, what I did the weekend before. In fact, the friend I was talking about earlier said, 'It's like time's lubricated,' which is an interesting metaphor given the physiological symptom of dryness. It's like it's much more episodic, you know. If you were to ask me what I was doing last weekend I'd probably struggle to remember, and the weekend before. I'd have to probably go back and just have something to remind me what I was doing, whereas before I'd say, 'Oh, yes, November was the month that we did these things.' It's all very much more discrete and when an event is over, it's sort of over – it's not entirely *lost* but I need pegs to remember. So, that feels very different and slightly scary really.

I know that often at work I have a sense of being like an old person who can't kind of get their act together, especially around technology! There're the standard things of not being able to find words, not being able to remember names, all of those sorts of things. I think I do rail against it and I think that probably makes it worse. I get very frustrated and feel like it shouldn't be happening. And, yes, I worry about it. I hope I'm going to recover some of it or maybe this is ageing, just ordinary ageing. So, yes, that, for me, has been a shock.

I mentioned earlier the 'change of life'. The other thing I've just noticed, and some of this is positive and some of this is just surprising, is that I feel very differently about ambition, career ambition and that sort of thing. For a lot of my time I was always looking to develop the next thing, you know. I did my psychotherapy training in my forties, and within that there's lots of scope to keep on learning, and I find I just don't feel as ambitious now. I kind of settle for what I've got which is, I think, a positive thing actually. You know, on one level it's kind of content, but I hardly recognise myself in a way. It feels very different. I don't know how much of that is post-analysis as well.

Also, the other change of age is having an elderly parent who is more vulnerable and needs more attention, but I find myself feeling that's what I want to be doing whereas when I was a bit younger, I'd have thought of it as a bit of an inconvenience. I'd have thought it was getting in the way of what I wanted to do whereas now I think – no, no, this is life, this is how it is. I think it's a kind of positive thing, though strange. I think along with it is a recognition of mortality and a time of wanting to consolidate really – there's less time left than there is behind.

But I wouldn't want to make it sound like it's all calm and Buddhist-like. There're certainly my mood swings that are quite intense. I think I've always been quite ready to get frustrated when things don't go right and I'd got better at managing that, but now I can get into quite a lather about things which I think only my partner will see. She just puts it down to the menopause, very generously.

I do also get into quite extremes of feeling and I think some of it is hormonal because it does remind me of when I had my periods and pre-menstrual tension. It's kind of the menopausal equivalent of that and perhaps more intense sometimes. I have also recently had some depression. When I was younger, in my twenties, I did have periods of depression and my analysis really helped. I haven't experienced real depression for a long time, just ups and downs. But recently I've had a few times when I've woken up and felt very bleak, the more negative side of contentment actually. Just feeling emptier, more barren and sterile and those kinds of feelings. Again, I think this may be menopausal. It's that sort of – what's it all about? What have I achieved? I've got no creativity, and all that. It doesn't linger, but I'm aware of it in a way that I hadn't been for a while.

The other thing I haven't mentioned is *anxiety*. I never really saw myself as a particularly anxious person. I've always seen myself as a fairly adventurous person who tends to be optimistic, but I am more anxious and sometimes in a quite unspecified way. You know, just a general anxiety and I've realised that I need to find something to fix it onto – to hang it on. I notice that, for example, when we had all the building work for the house going on and a lot to think about, I was less anxious about work because I had another anxiety, but when the building finished the anxiety about work returned.

The only other thing that I can think of – something more physiological – is that I've stopped having smear tests because it was just too painful. Smear tests were always painful for me (my womb is in a quite a hard to reach place), but since the menopause after several efforts I got referred to a Women's Unit to see a consultant and she said, 'Well, maybe there comes a point at which you have a balance up whether or not it's worth it.' So, that's a risk I carry and another reminder that there's stuff going on. I've never been very interested in HRT, I've always seen it as, 'let's just get through it', but, I suppose, if any of the symptoms were much more severe, I could see why people would have it.

So, it's certainly a passage to be negotiated and I do think – when will it end? Is there an ending? How do you know when you're through it? It *does* end, doesn't it? Plenty of people will have come out the other side.

KAREN

It has never felt like the end of my youth. I feel at the height of my life.

I've had a very easy menopause. I think I've already gone through my menopause. I'm fifty-one now. My last period was probably, I don't even remember, I think about three years ago and since then I have not had any bleeding, I've had very few hot flushes and I've only noticed a little bit of an increase in body temperature, particularly when I meditate – interestingly, that's when I'm most aware of it. I don't actually know whether those are hot flushes, but I do sometimes feel a sort of heat rising in my body, and then after a short moment it passes away. It happens mainly at the beginning of meditation, but not every day. This has happened particularly this year – these heat waves flowing through my body, but they have not been particularly unpleasant, though very noticeable. I do remember very well when this has happened and each time, I would ask myself, 'Uh, might this be a hot flush?', because I didn't know what one felt like.

I feel I've had a very easy menopause and it almost feels as though it happened without me noticing it. I'm very relieved that it's been so easy because my periods had been very painful, particularly in my forties, though not at all painful when I first started having them. I think I was about maybe thirteen when I was bleeding for the first time and from then onwards until my mid to late thirties I hardly had any pain, very little bleeding, no pre-menstrual signals. It was very regular but then something happened, and I don't know what that was, but some change in my body in my mid to late thirties. From then until when my periods stopped three years ago, I had excruciating period pain for the first three days of my period and very heavy bleeding. It's interesting that I had no pain at all before that age, but then a lot of pain and again no pain at all during menopause.

I also have not noticed any mood swings at all which I know some of my female friends talk about and often say, 'Oh, it must be my hormones.' I have not had any mood swings, as such, that I would put down to menopause or, you know, changing hormone levels. I've not been to the GP because of anything happening with menopause or me thinking 'Oh, this is menopause or hormones."

After a short pause Karen said she would like to add a little more:

When it became clear that I didn't seem to have periods anymore and no pain ... ah, it was such a relief. Maybe because my menopause hasn't been very pronounced it hasn't had such an impact because it's been so unnoticeable. It has never marked the beginning of a new chapter in my life or the end of my youth. It has never felt like the end of my youth.

Actually, I feel at the height of my life. This is to do with my spiritual life, which is very nourishing for me, inspiring and helpful. I feel I am in a kind relationship to myself, others and the world. And in terms of my work and my contribution to the world I feel at the height of my life because I'm now able to contribute to the world in the way I want to contribute which I hadn't been ten years ago or even five years ago. So, I'm really quite pleased about my age.

I feel grounded and confident in myself. I am enjoying my life and feel rather positive about life despite being fifty-one, or *because* of it! Having gone through menopause makes me think: 'OK, it's just a natural development in my being a human being, I guess, and part of maturing as a woman.' I see it positively as part of moving into a different phase in my life. I have the feeling my fifties will be more fruitful and enjoyable than my forties because I know so much better what I want and my place in life.

AYESHA

At a fundamental level, I don't want to get old. Yes, that's the truth and I know it's not an admirable or helpful attitude, but it's the way it is for me if I'm totally honest.

I know this is about the menopause but the first thing I want to say – and it's not unrelated – is that I find this whole ageing thing much more of a struggle and far, far more conflictual than I ever would have believed of myself. It's the physical signs of ageing that I'm struggling with – and this is the bit that surprises me.

Throughout my life –since my early twenties – I've kicked against the unrelenting and oppressive focus on girls' and women's looks, but over the last few years it's become quite an issue for me – my appearance I mean. I hate seeing my face age and feel like it's doing so at a rapid rate. I can feel unhappy and preoccupied with it, and then totally ashamed of myself for allowing it to affect me so much. I thought that being a feminist and very *pro-women* all my adult life would get me through this stuff pretty much unscathed – well, not exactly unscathed, but that it would provide me with enough of a framework or a context in which to consider these things. It hasn't though – well not so far – and this both shocks and disturbs me.

Yes, I think about the endless pressure that's put on women and their appearance and feel really strongly about it, but then in myself I feel that I've succumbed to it, got caught up in it. And I don't want to. I want to *refuse* it. It's like my thoughts and wiser perspectives are drowned out by these other mindlessly strong feelings – it's awful and feels so un-feminist (if there is such a word). Being a feminist has been an important part of my life and it's failing to see me through! Of course, I guess most people balk occasionally at their own ageing and that is probably ordinary, but the strength of my feelings is far too great and feels so unlike myself. But, maybe I can put these out-of-character and intense feelings down to the Menopause? Also, come to think of it, it only started when I was about forty-six which, I've read, is about the age when perimenopause often begins. I don't really know how to account for myself otherwise. Apparently, Simone de Beauvoir found her ageing looks terribly difficult too, so at least I'm in good company ...well, possibly.

I remember when I was young, probably in my mid to late twenties, I heard someone on the radio speaking about 'laughter' lines and 'thinking lines' on a woman's face, and she talked about them as being a sign of life and having lived. I thought it a great and insightful thing to say, and quite playful too. I remember her also commenting on the idea that ageing skin was primarily down to sun exposure. To this she said something like – who'd want to be so preoccupied with their skin and its eventual ageing that they'd miss out on the pleasures of swimming in the sun and feeling the lovely warmth of the sun on their face and body? I was really struck by her and remember thinking how I'd like to be the person saying those things. Her emphasis was entirely on life and living. Now, I think to myself, 'What's the hell's happened to me?' Why can't I use that now, apply it to myself?', because it's so unarguably true.

Anyway, more specifically about my menopause – that's why I'm here speaking to you after all. I'll be fifty-one this year and I think I'm perimenopausal as I still have periods. They're getting a bit more erratic now, but I still get them very frequently. I actually sometimes get them more often – I can now get a period every two and a half weeks or every two months. I didn't realise this was a symptom until I mentioned it to a friend, and they said the same thing.

I get some of the typical stuff going on, but not in a major way – well not yet anyway. It's mainly disturbed sleep, which is a pain, but not dire, touch wood. Also, like I said earlier, I have much stronger and sort of irrational emotions – not that emotions are rational, but what I mean is that I can't always explain them or connect them with anything that's going on. I can cry at the drop of a hat – I've always been a bit of a cry-er but to a far less degree. Also, I can get upset in an existentialist sort of way which is sometimes quite distressing. I've heard my friends say this too. I suppose this very real process of ageing confronts us with both our lives and our deaths. This is hard to think about though, more positively, it fires me to keep going and remember I'm not old, even if I think I look a lot older!

What else? I've not had any hot flushes, though I can wake up feeling quite hot and have to fling the sheets off for a while, but no sweats. A thing I don't like is that I can feel a lot more sluggish, a bit like having a long or permanent PMT – that sort of heavy, lethargic, washed-out feeling. It's hard to feel bright and breezy a lot of the time, or to wake up feeling properly refreshed. It's like in my spirit I feel youthful, yet my body *cruelly* reminds me I'm not and lets me down – very annoying.

Also, I'd say there's definitely a change going on in my sex life. It's like the usual ability to climax just doesn't happen. Well, no, that's not quite right, it does happen quite a lot of the time, but not nearly so easily or reliably. It's really very weird – I feel all the same sensations in my body that would normally lead to orgasm, but then … just nothing happens. It feels like something's been disconnected, switched off. It's very odd. (By the way, if this is a bit graphic don't put it in, but maybe other women will find it useful to read?)

I started my periods quite early, when I was twelve. I thought that because of that I might have a been a bit further on with the menopause by now. This isn't based on any evidence or reading or anything, just a feeling I had. I guess I thought we probably menstruated for about forty years so I should be about done by now. Perhaps there's no correlation whatsoever regarding these two things – I don't know, I've not looked into it.

A good few of my friends who are my age have either totally stopped their periods by now or have them far less frequently than me. In one way, it'd be nice to not have to bother with the hassle of periods and the discomfort, but I feel I don't really want *not* to have them. It's so clearly a blatant sign not only of the loss of youth, but also the loss of one of the things that makes me a woman. Having said that, the menopause is another thing that makes me a woman, I suppose. Lose one, gain one!

It can be a bit maddening, too, that men don't have to go through it. Well, there is a male menopause, but I don't think it's as trying or powerful for most men as it can be for women. Having said that, maybe I'm being a bit unfair and ignorant – some men may have a bad time, but just don't speak out about it. I don't really know enough about a male equivalent of menopause; I've just heard bits about it over the years.

Putting my personal struggles about my ageing face aside for a moment, I find the whole issue of women and ageing per se can make me very frustrated. Well, more than that, it can be infuriating. It's such a huge deal imposed upon women and can put us under a lot of pressure. It's just not fair. When I was thinking about this before coming here to talk to you, I was tempted to blame men and our male dominated culture for doing the imposing and offending, but I actually don't think it's just about that, by any means.

I've been thinking a lot about women and a certain competitiveness between women. Maybe this has its origins in patriarchy, I'm not sure. What I mean is that *women* can put a lot pressure or inject ill feeling, often inadvertently, on each other about their looks or physique. It's a sort of aggression, I guess. I don't really use the term 'passive aggressive', but some may call it that. As a woman's woman it took me a long time to allow myself to recognise this as a *thing* that goes on. I'm probably not being that clear but what I mean is if, for instance, I listen out in the street – or wherever – there is so much conversation and remarks between women about other women's looks, including stuff about ageing. You don't need to go far to hear it. I feel incredibly irked about this, and sad really. It gets to me most if I'm in the company of women who are saying things like, 'She really doesn't look her age', 'She's great for her age', 'Her skin is so amazing – she could pass for thirty-five'; 'You'd never guess she was fifty!', and so on, and so on. I know these things are meant as compliments and can feel like a boost, but what gets to me is that at that moment when such comments are made is that the woman *becomes* her looks – she is entirely perceived in terms of her appearance for that moment. It's like a constant reminder or even insistence between women that our looks are valid material for conversation and occupying our head space, but surely it's all just so banal and empty? Where do such conversations go? Where's the interest? Isn't it all just so boring and stultifying? And I *hate* the fact that I get caught up in it, embroiled in such nonsense. It's very powerful and painfully affecting.

Of course, far more offensive things are said too, and all sorts of disgraceful and damaging words given to women regarding the way they dress and present themselves. I'm talking now, though, about the daily, sort of accidental sexist and ageist comments. It brings to mind the recent book, 'Everyday Sexism'I have one friend who will mention her age or other women's' ages and appearances every time we meet. Women who call themselves, and are, feminists aren't immune to any of this, including myself of course. It seems to be so deeply ingrained that I think it's really hard to know how to fight it and oppose it – it's a competitiveness and sort of oppression that I'm sure we could all do without. I heard a woman saying her mother had gone on HRT to preserve her looks. Well, I don't know what to make of that really – it certainly says a lot about the importance of looks to her. I wish this could change for women somehow or other. I'm not blaming women, but I think women need to be more aware of it if anything is going to change in this sphere. It's not really talked about much in my experience.

Back to the menopause – I guess I don't know how it will pan out for me. I'm probably in the early stages and already finding the symptoms a bit of a bother, to be honest. That probably sounds really feeble as they aren't too bad on the scale of it. However, I think I'll talk to my GP about HRT at some point – just to see if it's an option to have on the back burner in case things get worse or too hard to manage. I'd want to know the ins and outs of it, the side-effects, how it was monitored etc, and try not to be fobbed off in a ten-minute appointment. I think some women see

HRT as a cop out or 'not doing it properly', but does it really matter if it helps? Well, it doesn't to me. It makes me think of when women talk – well brag – about their 'natural' birth compared to a medicalised one, let alone a caesarean. Again, it's a case of women putting other women under pressure, giving each other a hard time.

What else? Well, my main point is, on the one hand, I'd like to accept ageing and the menopause as processes that are part of my life as a woman but, at the same time, I'd really rather not go through them and would like things to stay the same! At a fundamental level, I don't want to get old. Yes, that's the truth and I know it's not an admirable or helpful attitude, but it's the way it is for me if I'm totally honest.

Maybe if we, as a society, valued old age more I might feel differently – who knows? My challenge is to find more of an accommodation with it and I hope that when I read your book and hear other women's voices it will help me.

Anyway, all that I've said is a bit of a jumble and all over the place, but that's where I am with it all at the moment. I would like to get to an easier place with it all and feel more harmonious. I'd like to grow older gracefully or, even better, disgracefully! Maybe saying it all here will be the first step in doing this … let's see.

Oh, just one last thought – I wonder how often are men intercepted in shopping centres and offered face and eye creams for their age lines?

LINDA WRITES

*There were no warning signs as to when I may have
sudden and intense periods of anger, sadness and sometimes
elation. I really didn't know who I was.*

When I finished treatment for breast cancer in 2006, aged
forty-five, I didn't realise that one of the side effects of
chemotherapy would be the early onset of the menopause.
Having had surgery, chemo and radiotherapy I was
obviously relieved to be 'coming out the other side', but my
hormones had a nasty trick up their sleeves. I was
menopausal – very quickly and pretty extremely.

I experienced nauseating and frequent hot flushes, some
like a wave starting at my feet and working up through my
body. They couldn't be ignored and the ones at night
interrupted my sleep for a number of months. As I had had
to have a hysterectomy at forty-two, because of fibroids, I

wasn't having periods, so it was hard to see if there was any monthly cycle relating to the menopausal symptoms. The mood swings were the pits, and thinking of, let alone having, sex was extinct.

The treatment that I'd had from the NHS for breast cancer had been both personal and attentive, but after the medical treatment it felt that I'd been spat out the other side and had to deal with these extreme menopausal symptoms myself.

Being youngish, my friends weren't really having the same hormonal changes, so I didn't really have a peer group to share things with and get support from. There is possibly the feeling that having survived the cancer treatment you're OK, but the menopause that followed left me emotionally and physically down.

As the mum of a nine-year old boy at the time there was guilt about not being able to look after him properly when I was having treatment, but I then questioned if I was a fit mother when the mood swings kicked in because of hormonal imbalances. There were no warning signs as to when I may have sudden and intense periods of anger, sadness and sometimes elation. I really didn't know who I was.

I asked for medical advice about the menopausal symptoms. HRT wasn't an option because I have a blood disorder which means that it clots too readily, and I have a history of having small strokes. HRT, apparently, can lead to strokes, so it wasn't going to be appropriate for me.

With hindsight I could have followed up getting more support, but I was knackered and pretty nuts, and not really able to disentangle the physical and emotional effects of the cancer treatment from the menopausal symptoms.

On the plus side this extreme menopause only lasted about 8 months – I didn't kill anyone, and I gradually stopped having about five different emotions in a minute. The hot flushes became more manageable and I stopped going puce in meetings.

Told you it was a horror story, but now a mellow fifty-seven-year-old with no menopausal symptoms. Still a bit grumpy sometimes, but I usually know why!

LOUISE

I just like to act on the spur of the moment sometimes. I like to jump on the train and go off to the seaside. Now if you're feeling like a sack of ten potatoes you can't even move.

Menopause – horrible, absolutely horrible. I know there are women out there saying we should celebrate it all. Sorry, but no! I'd rather just not have it, thank you very much.

I'm the kind of person who likes to run around town, I've always been like that. When I was younger I was an athlete, so I'm very, very active. And what I find with the menopause is that it's just slowed me down, in a bad way. All these hot flushes that I just get all of a sudden, you know, from the neck up, are just so debilitating. It really, really is and I feel really quite embarrassed about it as well.

I remember once I was on telly doing a programme talking and then all of a sudden – because it happens more in the evening and at night – I could just feel the heat coming up, like I was cooking in the oven from the neck up and then there was like a waterfall of sweat. There was nothing I could do about it. I just sat there feeling very embarrassed and continued talking. The person who was presenting it – I'm not using any names, but is well-known – was like, 'Oh my god, are you alright Louise? Are you alright?', you know.

I tell you what then did happen, one of the young production team – when we came on again – came over and she gave me a tissue and she said, 'See if you can wipe your brow.' She was *so* unsympathetic, and I wanted to say to her, 'Actually I'm on the menopause,' and stuff. It actually kept me away from telly for a bit because I thought, 'This is what's going to keep happening.' Then one day I thought, 'No, this is a nonsense, this is rubbish. This is part of the world I live in, part of the job that I do and I'm just going to do it.' So, when I go to do my shows, I just tell them, 'I'm menopausal,' straight off, you know, and there's no drama.

But it was really interesting that it was a young woman who said that to me, it wasn't one of the young male production team. It was her, and she was very unsympathetic.

As I said, I don't feel that I have as much energy as I had. I just like to act on the spur of the moment sometimes. I like to jump on the train and go off to the seaside. Now if you're feeling like a sack of ten potatoes you can't even move.

I'm alright at the minute because I think that some of my symptoms are sort of going – the women in my close family get menopausal in the late forties and then it's all done by fifty-three and stuff. One of the worst things though is the sleeping. Can't sleep! The tossing, the turning, oh my word. But the madness going on in your head as well because you're getting more and more and more frustrated. And I thought, 'How am I going to deal with this?' So, what I used to do if it got to half past one or two o'clock and I still wasn't sleeping, I'd just get up and make a cup of tea, watch some Netflix or Game of Thrones, gasp a couple of times and try to sleep. Usually the second time round I can sleep. I never have a full night's sleep, I always wake up, but I don't mind if I wake up and turn over and go back to sleep. But that's been terrible.

Another thing that has been terrible are the moods, you know. I don't call them moods actually. This is how I'd describe it – I wake up some days, and I had one of these yesterday, feeling like the world was coming to an end, and because I feel like the world's coming to an end there has to be an order to everything. I don't want to say it's OCD because people who have OCD have a real, real condition, but it's like I've got a couple of little tics. We've all got these little tics. So, every now and again if things are chaotic in my life, I have to go up to my office and tidy it up, particularly the rug in the middle of the room. It sounds really odd, because I'm not into symmetry – Feng-Shui, nothing like that – but it's got to be nice and centred and if it is, I feel nice. It's a bit weird, I know, a bit odd!

So, yes, I have those days when I feel the world is coming to an end, I feel so anxious, I feel like I want to cry. Yesterday, I felt the whole day like I wanted to cry and as soon as I saw poor L, my partner, instead of saying, 'Oh, good morning', I just glared at him and was ready to have a go at him about any silly thing. Poor bloke, he's done sod all wrong and I'm roaring away. It doesn't last the whole day – it'd be half an hour with him, but the whole thing lasts the whole day in my head. I've woken up today feeling, 'Wow! It's great, it's fabulous'. I don't know if that also is connected to the weather because the weather yesterday was grey and overcast, and I felt like that.

The plus of the menopause is no more periods – weh-hey! I've had a sub-total hysterectomy. You know, I don't like those women things if I'm honest. I don't have kids. My womb hangs out with me, it's nothing more than that. This is not the word which we use anymore, but the word that people would have used to describe me when I was growing up was a Tomboy. I was adventurous, active and that's kind of how I've always been. So, all these female things … I know other people want to celebrate them and I think, 'Good for you and you should'. We shouldn't be ashamed but, I'm sorry, I can't be dealing with it.

I tell you what, I thought because I hadn't had kids – this is really silly – that I'd get a really mild menopause. I think actually I have had a mild one, but I just thought a lot of the symptoms would just pass me by, like really it must be connected to something to do with people having a kid, you know.

Because I'm somebody who likes to be in control of my life, of myself and what I'm doing, the idea that I can't be in control of my emotions when I'm feeling so anxious is just really, really scary. As I said, yesterday I just felt like crying all the time. I didn't do it – maybe I should try actually doing it because then I'd think, 'What the heck am I crying about?'

I'm a real problem solver, if there's a problem let's see if we can sort it out. I used to be a teacher, it's all the whole teaching and learning thing – let's move forward – a bit of Vygotsky, you know. So, another big part of me was thinking, if I'm hot at nights, sweating, what can I do? And I don't sweat like other people do when they say they're drenched and stuff, I'm just alarmed by it. So, I was going all over the internet and looking at forums, but I didn't want to become part of a forum. One of the big breakthroughs for me was a *Chillow pillow* – they're really common now but back then when I bought one it wasn't so common – and that was lovely, so finding little bits and pieces that help has been really good.

I just try not to think about it. I just hope it goes away as soon as possible. It's not something I enjoy. And it's *definitely* not something I want to celebrate.

ELAINE WRITES

Breaking the glass ceiling

I knew something was 'wrong' when I broke down in
tears mid-music lesson, sobbed, then had to pull myself
together, go home and cook dinner for some friends. I
was about 42.

Not long after, while walking down the street, I stopped
in my tracks. I don't remember the symptoms (probably a
prickly neck), but that was the moment it dawned on me:
it's the menopause.

From about the age of 40, I had stopped sleeping through
the night – unheard-of for me – but only years later did I
realise that this too had been an early signal.

I largely escaped hot flushes. All I remember is a horribly prickly neck and feeling absolutely 'all over the place'!

Saying I felt 'stressed', 'anxious' and 'agitated' doesn't seem quite accurate. I felt like I'd never felt before, and the movie image that always came to mind was the scene of the villain falling off the top of a building and crashing through glass ceilings below.

My much older French friend kept me sane by being there to explain what was happening to my body. I remember thinking: why can I be in this position and in such a state of ignorance?

I did talk to my mum, but she just said her periods stopped abruptly at about 40, with no side-effects, or none that she remembered.

I took some Japanese soy product, but never considered HRT.

I felt the change was going to happen to your body some time somehow, so why fight it? (My French friend tried to come off HRT at nearly 70 and was so 'lost' and agitated that she had to start taking the pills again almost immediately.)

I did, however, go on the pill in the early days. This helped until one week I ran out and wasn't able to get a repeat prescription immediately. The fallout was sudden and dramatic. This was the time I really did fall through the glass ceiling.

The plunge in hormone levels triggered a few days of utter blackness and for the one time in my life I could look into the pit that is depression. I felt there was a chemical imbalance in my brain and only readjusting it would 'fix' me. No amount of reassurance, distractions, exercise, healthy food would work. Going back on the pill soon resolved the problem.

On another occasion when I felt wobbly (not pill-related), a friend turned up on my doorstep with a goody bag – chocolate, wine, video – and that was a welcome distraction and delight!

For me, the early years of the menopause was also a time of 'urgency', a time of hormones wanting a last hurrah … but that is another story.

KALLY

I like to be reminded that nature is bigger than us.

I guess initially I would say that it feels like the *unknown*, and I don't know if that's because it happens to women or because we're reliant on women of our mothers' generation to report back to us. I think is quite often the case with that generation, and definitely in my case, that it's just all untalked about. It was like that with periods, so we talked to peers.

It really *is* unknown in that it's so different for everyone. You don't know how long it's going to last; you've got no kind of map, but it just feels like there should definitely be more information out there.

Now, my personal experience is that I don't know if I've had it or not. For about six months I was quite bad with hot flushes and then my periods just stopped when I was about forty-nine or fifty. So, I don't know if I just got off really lightly or if that was just the perimenopause and that the full-on thing is still to happen. I don't really think of myself as being very mature, so I can't see why I would have had it early. I'm not a kind of 'grown-up, early' person, if you know what I mean?

So, I thought I'll stop drinking so much because then when it really comes it might not be so bad – it's all this kind of self-medication and unknown, but anyway I didn't. I just started drinking more! I then had a massive period after I'd had a smear test, so I don't know where I'm at really which is crazy when you think about it, isn't it?

What have I learnt? I've Googled things – thank god for Google. I've talked to friends and watched the Mariella Frostrup programme. Something I didn't realise until watching that programme is that I think you do have some control over, for example, the hot flushes. Before that, I thought it was just something that happened to you and you had no control over it whatsoever – it felt like it just came from nowhere. But when they had the group that went to the therapist, after that I thought, 'Oh, god, maybe.' And I did begin to notice that when I was in a stressful situation the hot flushes were definitely worse. If I was stressed at work they were definitely worse, for sure.

For example, one time I met with a friend for lunch and the waiter came to take our order, and she said, 'I'm having a hot flush,' and I said, 'Oh my god, so am I.' So, we were thinking, 'Why are we? Why are we both having a hot flush?" and then it was, kind of, 'Let's analyse it'. I don't know, I think it's trying to make sense of it and trying to take control of it rather than being a by-stander to it.

It's our bodies that it's happening to for god's sake. I think that we were both feeling a little a bit nervous. It sounds silly, because I wouldn't have said I was nervous about a waiter coming and taking an order, but I think I am a little bit. You know that kind of thing if someone is being subservient, it's a little bit of an uncomfortable feeling.

So, it did make me realise that we can have *some* control over it. At the moment things are a bit stressy at home and I'm waking up early feeling hot, so it definitely seems to relate to how content and happy I am, for sure, which I'd had no idea of before.

The other thing on the programme – thank god for that programme – was that Mariella Frostrup was having HRT, wasn't she. Personally, I would try and avoid taking any medication, just because I don't – it's the way I am. My kids aren't immunised. I tried to have natural births. I don't go near the doctor if I can possibly help. We're quite squeamish in our house, but also I just think, 'Don't mess with nature.' If nature can do it on its own, as soon as you start intervening things can go wrong, in my mind. Although, obviously, if I had cancer or a heart-attack or whatever, I'd be straight down to A&E.

And I'm not evangelical about it. But, anyway, she – Mariella Frostrup – was having HRT, and her gynaecologist, who obviously had a bit of a vested interest in keeping her on her books, was saying to carry on with it indefinitely, forever, potentially. This really shocked me because I've always thought the menopause was something that you went through for an unknown period of time – six months or ten years – and then you're over it. So, yes, that was a bit of a shock.

And everyone does say that when you're out of it, it's amazing, like you're just much less anxious and freer and so on. Well, I don't know, because I'm not there. Personally, though, I like a bit of up and down. I don't have any great dream for everything to be just quite calm and on a level. I'm more of an either full-on or full-off kind of person.

I don't know what else to say really. You see, I don't think about it that much at the moment. I haven't really noticed a massive, kind of, out of control emotional thing – maybe I just *always* am! I think I'm always a bit of a kind of nutty person in my head. I don't know if there's any difference, though I was expecting there to be.

I suppose that's the thing, as well, the more you know the more you're looking for things – it's kind of like reading a medical encyclopaedia, I suppose. I guess I'm trying to not make too much of a big a deal of it.

I feel reluctant, though, to say that, because it's a thing that happens to women and it *is* a big deal, and I do think if it happened to men it would be dealt with completely differently. And for some people who have twenty flushes an hour for ten years, say, it would take over your life. Touch wood, for me, that hasn't been the case and I don't want to make it a really big deal if it doesn't need to be.

Also, there's that kind of thing of people who say, 'She's a menopausal woman.' Well, fuck right off actually. It's not an insult, is it? It's not something to be laughed at.

Emotionally, I think, it's a weird and unknown time of life anyway for a lot of women. You know, the kids are gone, the parents start dying, your relationship changes. With these things thrown in I'm feeling different emotionally anyway. Possibly hormonally too, but possibly also because all these other things have been chucked at us.

It'd be great, though, if that was it for me. I don't know though. I guess the other thing to say is that I don't know how to find out. I don't know if I *can* find out. It seems all I can do, as I've said, is take control of it and go with it to an extent, but I don't actually know if I *could* find out. I'm not a doctor person, so I'm not going to start going for blood tests. Even if I did, I don't know what I'd do with that information.

But it is a weird thing isn't it, to have this thing happening to you and your body that you haven't really got a lot of control over and it's for an indefinite amount of time? I guess, as well, though, there's a weird side of me that actually also quite likes that – I like to be reminded that nature is bigger than us.

You know like when you have a baby, when you're pregnant, it's like, 'My body is doing this thing.' We get books and read and find out everything that we possibly can, but our bodies just get on with it. I think that's just amazing. It *is* amazing isn't it? You know, like when you look at the ocean and you think, 'Oh my god, the ocean is big.' So, I do *like* the fact that it's a bit of the unknown and just a reminder that there's this other massive thing going on that's more than us.

Oh, and one last thing to say relating to the nature issue, my daughter M's periods and mine were in sync when she was at home and the only time I have a glimmer of a period now is when she's at home. Amazing!

SHALMA

***You can get weepy, feel very down, feel like you just
want to cry. You don't know why, but you feel like you
just want to cry***

I don't know where to start talking about these sorts of
things …

I had really itchy skin on my body, all over the place. It
wasn't a rash, as such, it was just this completely horrible
itch all the time. Then I had sleepless nights, and noticed
mental and physical differences, I suppose. I didn't really
put it down to anything and then it was only afterwards that
I spoke to a doctor and she actually said it could be the
menopause, or the onset, the perimenopause.

You can get weepy, feel very down, feel like you just
want to cry. You don't know why, but you feel like you

just want to cry. I just put it down to depression. The things that I didn't really experience were the hot flushes. I think they are sort of coming now, in a way. Even on a really cold day I can find myself, you know, very sweaty and hot and think it's probably that.

Once I knew this is what it was, I didn't think it would affect me the way it did. I think that it took a while to put it into perspective – my whole personality as a woman. You do feel this loss that you're not a whole person anymore and it's quite sad, in a way, to feel that. You feel like you're sort of dried up, though it is literally like that, I guess.

Well, I've got children and grandchildren. You don't ever think when you're going through your life that one day it is going to come to a stop and you're not going to be a woman anymore. You're made to feel – well some people make you feel – like you're not a person anymore, and it's amazing how you can just be tossed aside. Literally it's like you've bought something, and you've used that thing up and you can then throw it away. I'm talking about the physical side of things. It's family members that can sometimes have that effect on you. They can make you feel like that without having *any* clue what's really happening to you, to your body, what you're going through or any understanding at all. It makes you feel like, 'Oh my god'.

I can't really blame anybody. My husband doesn't know what's happening to me, and even if he did, he wouldn't really understand it. He's made throw-away comments and they have really affected me – it's too personal to really say what. Like I said, I could explain it like the empty drink carton can be just thrown away. You've had your day, you've had your youth, so now you're not really much use to anybody. That affects me a lot.

There are not a lot of people who are aware of it in our community, in the community as a whole. I'm not just putting it down to the Bengali community. There's not much information or talk about it. It's like no one talks about this sort of thing unless like now with you, on a one-to-one. I don't really think about it unless I'm reading about it or hearing about it on TV or something, you know.

So, it'd be really interesting to know how other women have coped or how it was for them, you know, and what to expect because it's not like 'one size fits all' – it's not like that at all. Women are different, and our approaches are different, so how we cope with things like that are different, I guess.

I had this cloud, this distraction of having open-heart surgery and trying to recover from it, so that sort of took away most of my symptoms because I packaged everything together in one. It felt that everything going on in my body was due to my heart – I had a valve replacement. I put all my symptoms down to that one thing, whatever was because of the valve or the operation and recovery.

Emotionally, I felt unsupported and misunderstood. Nobody realises the fact that women at a certain age have these huge things happening to them and, as a result, all sorts of things come up. And it's not because they're feeling, you know, in a bad temper or being horrible – it's just that they're not having a good day and feeling really bad. I wanted to explain, especially to my daughter, but she didn't understand. We're very close, but I just didn't know how to explain to her because I didn't know how describe it myself at that time. I was very moody; I didn't really smile. At the time you don't understand what it is. Like I said, I had one explainer for it, it was all down to the operation. It wasn't. Maybe it did have some effect, but everything was made worse.

I guess if I was to change anything or be able to do anything again, it would be to have some kind of understanding in the family. In our community, though, it is one of the taboo subjects, nobody even knows about it. The menopause *is* something, but it's one of those things you couldn't talk about, even if you wanted to. But I would say, find somewhere like a women-friendly place where you can say what you're going through – your symptoms and all of that, and have a little chat if you're feeling really out of sorts. Just being supported I guess, would really help.

What's new to me at the moment, is that I've got some kind of late bleeding that can happen – a massive post-menopausal bleeding that's happened in one week. As a result, I'm going through all sorts of tests to see if it's not something more sinister. I've already been to the gynaecologist and they said sometimes it happens – you can get some spotting or bleeding or whatever. It still needs to be investigated and that's a worry because you think the worst. Anyway, I'll know at the end of the tests if it's just a normal process when going through the menopause.

It's good to be here now, you know. A couple of years ago it wasn't a such a good place. I think the one thing I would *really* like to emphasise is your partner. You know, I don't expect him to be aware, but maybe a GP could talk to them and say, 'Well, this is what's happening to your wife, or whatever, and this is what you need to be aware of.' Then they might be a little bit more sensitive and not be so cruel in some ways, like in the comments they make. They just make you feel you're a used rag doll or something, you know, just toss you aside like that and I think that's the worst feeling ever. That's taken a *huge* toll on me. I wanted to lash out, but then I thought, 'Well he doesn't know and even if I tried to explain it he wouldn't understand it', I don't think. So, that's been a huge thing for me.

We're heading into old age, and just because we're having menopause doesn't mean it's the end of us as women, as people. I think that what I've come away with is that we can't stop what happens to us – it's our body yet out of our control. Emotionally you can be made to feel that it is *your* fault, then your self-esteem goes completely down to zero. You're not a beautiful person anymore and then you don't feel like you want to make any effort anymore.

Those were the things that had me going for months and months and months. It took a lot of soul-searching and a lot of talking to people and hearing them saying, 'We know what you're saying' – that helps such a lot. It's like, finally, someone understands and that I'm not crazy.

Again, having this health distraction gave me something else to focus on otherwise I think I would have had a really, really bad time. I've been through quite a bit and, in a way, I'm relieved that it's over. I'm not bothered so much now because I know so much more about my body.

The feelings about my self-esteem and everything still get to me and I think my relationship with my husband has been affected by that. I think I'm still very cross with him and feel like he should have understood. Even though I know that there's no way he could – my expectation is that he should have. He should make allowances for the fact that this is something that I have no control over. I'm not young, you know, I'm not who I used to be. It's been a bit of a shock for him to see that I'm growing old. Age you can't stop. He should have been supportive because he's an older man, but it's sort of like, 'Oh, you're past your sell-by date,' you know. That's the attitude and the only way I can explain it. And there was a point where he actually did think of replacing me, I suppose. He talked about it; he didn't do it – all he could do was talk about it, like 'Well, you're no good. I'm just going to find myself a younger model who'll do this for me.' That is just the most amazingly cruel thing that I have experienced. If I put everything else aside that alone is very damaging for somebody's mental state. You think, 'What is it about me? I don't look *so* drastic, so what is it you're saying?' It took me years and years to come to that conclusion.

I think it is a cultural thing, or something. I didn't have to take on that blame of not servicing somebody in the way a twenty-year-old would, and all that. You don't have the same kind of drive and you don't feel that kind of need – you know, in the physical side of things. At the moment I am OK with not having the physical side – it doesn't bother me at all. I'm actually quite relieved!

I'm finding out about it more, learning about it. I go to see women and I ask questions. I'm coming to a place where I'm ok because I understand and I'm trying to become comfortable with it. You know, it's been a learning process for me, just as much as a process on my body, so I think I'm in a better place than I was a couple of months ago.

Shalma added after we stopped recording that she wanted it noting that she is currently getting the wheels in motion to set up a 'Well-woman' clinic where women can come and talk about their health. She sees this as the way forward.

.

TATIANA

Tulip

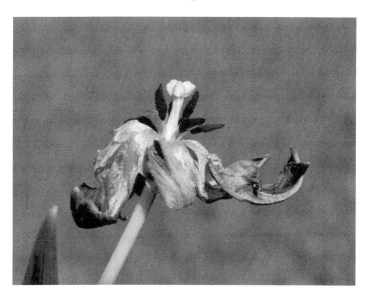

I took this picture in my garden. All the tulips were well gone, and it was time to cut the stems back. And here it was – the last one standing with a bended stem shrinking from dehydration. I could not stop looking at the way it gracefully spread its petals, holding on strongly to every few that were left. I thought that it was only when this delicate flower was bruised by elements from the outside, which dried it out and turned its exterior colour to dusty grey, that it began to shine from the inside.

SAMIRA

It's seen as though I'm not going through menopause properly – it's ridiculous. It's absolutely ridiculous.

There are two things: the first thing is that I'm an avid listener of *Woman's Hour*, and I would actually say that since I started listening to it, which was in 2010, that programme has really helped me. I wouldn't say emancipated me, but it did help me to get a perspective of what positions we take in relation to menopause, or what we get allotted by society.

And the other thing has struck me – with childbirth there is a kind of machismo, a female version of machismo, I don't know the word, 'femismo' maybe? I've always found that, in a funny sort of way, when I hear women talk about being in labour, they talk about it in a way that clearly they were suffering, but that it was also something heroic.

Like, you know, 'I did 27 hours, and I had …. and so on,' and you think, 'What the hell is going on?' Nobody talks really about how they feel, but, actually, it's like, 'I was able to endure this thing which lasted blah, blah, blah'. I have never had a child, so I can't really speak about that except for what I've heard other women say about it. Strangely enough though, I think there's something among women themselves where this heroism comes back into play with menopause.

But, then, it's like this tough talking of Theresa May saying, 'Just get on with the job.' What job? What does it *mean* 'get on with it?' What is it that you have to push away of yourself because it is too confronting to others? I think, 'Bullshit, let's stop doing that.' It's just not fair.

Some women have the luck that they don't have the hot flushes, and I was definitely one of them. However, I take HRT and I've been taking it for four years, five years since I was in menopause. The reason is that I was having too many physical problems. I couldn't sleep properly, my hair was thinning, and I also had vaginal issues – it was really painful. Now, of course, because of that *machismo*, similar to how many women are made to feel if they have a caesarean or don't breastfeed, it's seen as a cop out. It's seen as though I'm not going through menopause *properly* – it's ridiculous. It's absolutely ridiculous.

I think it is a different experience for everybody, and I don't think the brush off that you can get is fair for those women who have real problems with it.

I'm mystified why it is, but I think talking honestly about menopause is a problem and I think, actually, as I'm talking to you, that maybe it's a similar thing as to why people find it difficult to talk about death, or anything that has an ending. It's too confronting perhaps, and that is why the whole thing becomes, in a way, very secretive, a mythical situation – and it's such a shame. I find it such a shame. Does this ring a bell with you, do you know what I mean?

I've heard women, and men talking about women's looks *going*. Well, they don't go, but things *change* physically – is this seen as going or changing? In my work when I meet younger women, I actually say to them, 'Life gets much nicer after fifty. I am enjoying my life better now than I did when I was forty'. So, there's this thing about *the change* that is absolutely right.

I would say that what *does go* are the looks from certain men, in a certain way. Apparently, the gaze of a man is only on you, I don't know, until you're about forty. Isn't that ridiculous? But that's the way it is. So, that element does go, but I don't mind about that.

I was fifty-seven when I went on HRT and, indeed, the whole thing of statistics is confusing. For years, of course, I didn't dare to because of the so-called twenty per cent risk of developing breast cancer. The update on the statistics that were given in the Mariella Frostrup programme is something to take into account – it was very good, and I'd actually already heard. I'd heard because I have a new gynaecologist – they thought there was a growth in my womb, but it turned out to be nothing sinister and I had a little operation.

Anyway, first of all I had a male gynaecologist as there was a bit of a rush because my GP was getting nervous, and this gynaecologist said, 'Come back next week, take a couple of paracetamol and I'll do the procedure'. I was out on the street feeling overwhelmed and thinking, 'I really can't handle pain and taking a couple of paracetamol while he takes a biopsy – well, I don't think that's a good idea.' But the fact that this can be said – how can you say as a doctor, as a male doctor, that you can just get through this procedure just on paracetamol? And so, I thought, 'Well, I'll wait a bit and go to a gynaecological surgery and find a woman.' I'd heard good news about this particular doctor, and I explained that it was the idea of the pain that was making me terrified, and she said, 'Oh, no, it's fine, we have sedation, very mild sedation, but we have sedation.' She didn't make me feel ridiculous, nothing at all like that.

If only women could allow themselves this, but it is put on us partly by doctors, I think, and by each other – *women* put pressure on each other, and this only makes it harder, you know. The heroic aspect of menopause, the admiration of looking young.

This thing of 'women against women' – I don't know how to change it. Where I work a woman was advised to use her looks for her work – she *liked* that comment and told me proudly. I said, 'What, what?' This cannot be true. It's awful, it's depressing.

I have a sister who is very glamorous and very concerned with her looks and, I have to say, one of my biggest traumas was my sisters pointing at my breasts and making funny remarks, and also my mother did. I had a strange mother who made fun of everything. It's an odd thing I'm going to say, but I lost my mother when I was very young and, in a way, not having my mother has probably made it easier to come to terms with the menopause. I'm sure she would have said terrible things, but she wasn't there to say them.

So, the combination of having therapy which, to be very clear, I don't think you need to do. I don't think women need to do this just because of menopause – that would be ridiculous. But just the fact of being a bit more secure and at ease with myself has made it clearer to see how trapped you can get, and I don't want to be trapped in that way.

And the other thing is, my relationship with men is fine. I mean, if they're talking bullshit, I just don't go along with it. It's not that I ever thought I had to be part of their prey, but now knowing that I'm certainly *not* makes it far, far easier – that I have to say. If they start complaining, which a lot of men seem very good at in order to get attention, I just look away and I say, 'Oh, OK,' and I just stop listening until they're done and then I start listening again. I even say, 'Do you have to complain about this?' Their lives can be perfect, but they need so much attention that they need to complain, but now I'm just not interested. I can see that I can be a threat to men though because, in a way, I sometimes I catch them out for a certain vanity and sense

156

of entitlement. And, I can also sense it when I don't want to be part of certain things like not taking competitive work life very seriously. This is hugely threatening to men, hugely. That's what I really like about getting older and I'm enjoying it!

I can see, if anything, and this is for women and men, the idea of losing my partner as I get older can creep up on me. This is an element that has to do with life more than being a woman and menopause.

Some of the symptoms I've had – I got very angry at some stage, and perhaps this is maybe what I mean about the benefits of having therapy when menopausal. You can get some sort of understanding of a certain sort of self-dissatisfaction, under accomplishment or whatever. Therapy made it easier for me to come to terms with my life and understand some of what's happened in it and get to know the sorts of reasons that I might be angry.

I think also that because women are reflected back differently to men by society, there's this feeling of inadequacy about how to deal with stuff, and then this rage can set in. The menopause can bring on this feeling of inadequacy that many women experience anyway. That is such a shame because how do you deal with that? You need help. People need to talk about it. Programmes like *Woman's Hour* need to be talked about.

But, going back to talking about looks, certain things to do with looks *do* go in a certain way and the question is how far you go to try to get them back, or keep them, or do you just relax about it and let it go. I'm questioning myself about that – it's a hard one though, and hard to go through. It's complicated.

I think the medical world really needs to spend time learning and keeping up with knowledge and what is out there, and to explain properly what is going on and not brush it off. If we go to a doctor, they brush it off, maybe because they don't have the solution or don't know enough about it, or they think you're just making a fuss about nothing.

IMAN

I can't think of anyone who talks about this in my community. I'm from East Africa, of Indian origin, and moved to the West when I was very young.

What do I think of the menopause? I think it's horrible, and it's unfair. The hot flushes, the useless sleepless nights – they make you feel yucky and tired almost all the time. I feel like I'm paying time for having an easy ride in my younger days. I can't remember when it all started as it was gradual, but I know that it feels like it's been going on for a long, long time. It just *won't* stop. The menopause makes me feel out of control with my life. I can never be sure how I'll feel as I can never be sure whether I'll get enough sleep, or not.

The menopause – I mean why is there a 'pause' in 'menopause'? Nothing pauses, it just stops. Your period stops, your youthfulness disappears, but you carry on. As I said, it just makes me feel *so* out of control with my life.

What's the other thing about the menopause that I absolutely hate? I *hate* the fact that I feel constantly tired – that's all related to the lack of sleep, of course. I go through weeks of only having two or three hours of sleep per night, and then I'm *so* tired and crabby. All these symptoms, I feel, are because of the great 'pause'. It has a significant impact on my life, and the people around me.

I think I look older than I did, and I don't know whether it's because I've stopped dyeing my hair, or whether it's the menopause. I certainly feel older. When people give up their seats on the tube I kind of think, 'Uh, is it because I look really tired or is it because I look old?' Ageing just isn't something that we are prepared for. We're not prepared when we're growing up, and it's even worse for today's generation. Thinking back to my youth and comparing it to my daughters', I know the whole business about the body image and all that has gone so overboard.

Also, my mother didn't help. She never talked about how old she felt, or how she felt about her looks, or about her menopause. It makes it feel wrong, somehow, this process of ageing. I wish she had spoken now, you know.

In fact, I can't think of *anyone* who talks about this in my community. I'm from East Africa, of Indian origin, and moved to the West when I was very young. I don't know why we don't talk about the menopause or ageing – it's as if it's taboo. When I travel on the tube, I see a lot of older Asian women who have dyed their hair. I often ask myself why they don't go grey naturally, go white naturally. Is there something to be *ashamed* of in terms of ageing for that particular cultural group? I made a conscious decision not to dye my hair for that reason and I feel *liberated* for doing this. I am trying to be open and honest about the ageing process.

I believe it is important to talk about getting older so that it doesn't surprise us when it happens – it shouldn't feel wrong. We should be able to embrace it and celebrate it. We don't talk about it outside of the home. Also, it should be openly included and discussed in the context of equality, inclusivity and diversity – ageism is rarely part of such discussions.

I would love to talk to my daughters about ageing so that they can be better prepared, and it might not come as such a shock to them. But it's a catch-22, as they are overly conscious of their bodies and I don't like drawing attention to their physical looks. Maybe when they're a bit older and wiser I will.

I could do without the menopause. If that could be taken out of the ageing equation then it would be better. So, I guess when I think about the menopause I always think about ageing and, 'Won't it be fantastic when this is all over and I can really enjoy my elderly status?'

MARY WRITES

I enjoy being older – I don't have an empty nest to cope with, just a sea of opportunity that is not blighted by the monthly collapse.

I will start by saying that I am happier, spiritually and mentally now I have been through the menopause. It did create a 'change' for me, a new lease of life. I know, not the reaction of most.

I started menstruating early – around ten and a half – and from around sixteen onwards suffered with the most awful PMS. For three weeks before my period I was energetic and engaged in life, and then the collapse. For three days before my period started, I would be so exhausted and depressed I could hardly move. All I wanted to do was to sleep and turn my back on the world. This meant the world of work and interaction was so difficult that I sometimes failed to take part.

To get through this period I ate – usually sugar, and the desire for sweet treats seemed to outweigh any thoughts of healthy eating. This kept me in a cycle of being large and often 'out of it' for years. I remember trying to get some recognition of what was going on only to be told by a female doctor to, 'Stop reading stupid articles in the *Observer* supplement – this is a made-up condition for the middle classes.'

So, menstruation was harder than menopause. I had ablation in my forties, so the bleeding stopped, however, the PMS persisted. Then, yes, hot night sweats, UTIs and a short temper, but this was nowhere near as debilitating and demoralising as what had gone before.

I enjoy being older – I don't have an empty nest to cope with, just a sea of opportunity that is not blighted by the monthly collapse.

I take a very small vaginal dose of HRT now, tiny but it helps with the libido. That is in and out, not constant but healthy.

Most of the changes in my body I do not mind as I am fitter than I was before. I hate the grey hair, cannot wait for the silver, at which point I will cease to be blonde. I did not sail through the process but feel that this chapter, while uncomfortable, opened vistas for me rather than shutting them down.

PAULINE

Vertigo

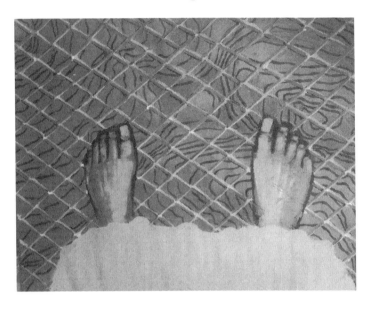

A dream state of

light-headed and dizzy

The feeling of 'jet lag' due to lack of sleep

from night sweats, hot then cold

Waking at night

and dreaming of standing outside in bare feet

JUDITH

I just find it deeply ironic that after so many years of being woken by young children, just at a time when they sleep late into the morning, I can't sleep beyond seven-ish – that's if I manage to go back to sleep after waking at four in the morning.

Well I think one thing that I've been thinking of a lot is actually how do you define menopause? Is it just a biological hormonal change or is it all the emotional and mental changes that go with being a certain age, and how do you disentangle those two things? I suppose what's occurred to me a lot, is whether when women go through an early menopause do they face the same sort of mental and emotional challenges as somebody who's say fifty, fifty-four or whatever? I just find that a very interesting question and would like to know more about it. I think a lot of what

I've gone through is about being a parent of two children who are almost grown-up themselves. If I wasn't doing that, if I perhaps didn't have children at all or if I'd had them a lot younger, would I still be going through a lot of those challenges about what happens next – where will I live, where will I work? Is that due to menopausal and hormonal changes or is it about a life change regardless of hormones and biology? So yes, I think that's one of the main things for me to grapple with – how do you define menopause?

In terms of biological change, I thought I was menopausal and then about a month ago I had a period which came out of the blue. I'd thought that was it for me, all finished! I'm fifty-four, but I've had two periods in about two years, both at times when I was incredibly stressed and physically very tired. One was when I had a really terrible tooth, I mean really bad – the worst pain I've had in my life actually, much worse than having a baby. I also had a period about a month or so ago when I was incredibly exhausted and stressed with my work situation, so I just thought that was interesting. The body is doing something at a time of high stress, and it's also like your body's having another go at releasing an egg or whatever, one last chance of fertility.

I certainly don't think I feel a sense of loss about losing fertility. If I hadn't had children, I'm sure I'd feel differently. I think having children and having gone through parenting, I don't feel that – those sorts of changes don't bother me so much.

The main symptom I've had is sleep disturbance, but again I think a lot of that is compounded by worries about work and money. There's no doubt though that probably since being perimenopausal my sleep's been more disturbed. I'll go to sleep fine actually, but then I'll wake up probably a few times a night. I won't stay awake for long until about four or five o'clock in the morning, and then that's the time when I'll often be awake thinking about things and my mind will start churning. I just find it deeply ironic that after so many years of being woken by young children, just at a time when they sleep late into the morning, I can't sleep beyond seven-ish – that's if I manage to go back to sleep after waking at four in the morning. It's really, really annoying, as well as very tiring because I like sleep, it's really important to me. I think I do wake up hot. I don't have the night sweats, luckily, but I do wake up a bit hot and have to have my window open even during the winter. So, the summer is not a good period in terms of sleep and getting over-hot and waking up more. If I've got a particularly busy time at work or worrying about things, then that just adds to it.

As I said, for me, there's been a lot of reflection about where do I want to go from here? You know, the future, those sorts of things. I don't know if that's just about menopause or whether that's just about the fact that I'm in my fifties. A lot of my peers are either reducing their hours at work or thinking about semi-retirement or retirement completely.

One of the things about work is that I identify as much older – lots of my colleagues are around thirty-ish, that's twenty-four years younger than me, a lot younger. And the people that are older than me are much more senior in

167

terms of their jobs. Now, that's partly because personal circumstances have meant I haven't gone up the career ladder, but also I don't know actually if ever I really *wanted* to. I have found it difficult, though, being a relatively junior member of staff. It's almost like my twenty-five years of work experience – because I've always worked even when I had children – doesn't matter, it's been completely discounted. So, these sorts of things I've found quite difficult, but, again, is that a menopausal thing or is it just being mid-life? I mean, the two you can't separate, can you?

So, yes, in terms of work there's that and I have tried recently to change my job, without any success yet. But part of not getting very far with looking for a new job is feeling, 'Is it my age?' I am very much a middle-aged woman and going into my mid-fifties, not even early fifties. Do potential employers, maybe on an unconscious level, not particularly want to have someone like me starting a middle range job? Maybe I'm seen as a little bit too independent with the experience I've got? Maybe they don't want somebody who's got all that experience. Maybe they want someone who is a bit younger, perhaps fresher, perhaps more energetic etc?

So, it's been quite a difficult experience having to face up to the fact that being older might mean that the changes you want to make, perhaps you can't in the way you could have done maybe ten years ago. There's a lot of difference between being in your early forties and early fifties. And again, the menopause has come in the middle of that, so …

It doesn't help too – and again I'm not sure if this is the menopause or if it's the years and years and years of working

– being a lone parent, doing all the parenting and all the bread-winning on my own. I feel a bit worn out, but is a biological change compounding that? Probably. I think most women say that menopause does make you feel more tired. Your energy levels do dip, I think. So many women in their early fifties will have had decades of working a lot or being a parent and getting quite worn out anyway, then hormonal change is going to add to that. So, I do feel really tired and maybe that also comes across at work. You sort of feel you're not as energetic as your younger colleagues, and you do think other people probably notice that. Certainly, in terms of my own self-esteem it definitely affects it – I can't cope with some of the things I used to cope with because my energy levels aren't as high.

I also think I get more anxious about things and, again, the two things are hard to separate. Do you get more anxious because you're tired and it is harder to cope with something if you're more tired, so being tired makes you more anxious? I think there's a vicious circle.

I should try to think of something positive about being mid-life. I think definitely one is going into a new era when my children are almost grown-up. That dependency on me is starting to dissipate now, a bit. I feel a greater sense of liberation about having the freedom to go and do the things that I want to do, even just going to the cinema and not having to worry about being at home that night and doing the dinner, or whatever. Hopefully, if I don't have to keep working as much as I do now, there will be more spare time for myself. But it's trying to find the way of being able to do that, being able to sort out my housing and employment so that income is good enough so that I can actually enjoy that spare time. And being cared for a little bit more – it's going to be more of a reciprocal relationship with the children. It's not just that I'm caring for my children, but that I might get cared for a little bit too, and that's already happening. My daughters look out for me and I feel a sense of being looked after more than I used to. So, that's definitely a positive side.

Having lots and lots of friends who are a similar age and going through similar things is helpful, although it is amazing how much people don't talk about it even with their close friends. I think it's partly because everyone seems to experience it differently, so it's quite a difficult thing to share. I mean, I've got friends whose periods stopped overnight at the age of forty-three and they never had any symptoms, or so it seems. And then other people obviously have hot flushes and quite difficult physical symptoms which I'm lucky I haven't had so much. I get very hot a lot, but no hot flushes, sweats and things like that. I've been lucky that I haven't had those physical symptoms, but I definitely have the tiredness and the cognitive stuff – a bit of a feeling of memory loss and I'm sure my concentration isn't as good as it used to be.

There's definitely something about feeling invisible, not really being noticed – not just when walking down the street, but in social situations and things. But is that a self-esteem issue? Is that something that's inside? Is it something dreamt up and then you're looking for it? Is it self-fulfilling? It's hard to disentangle all these things I think, and to really sort of analyse what's happening.

But, maybe it's inevitable at a period in your life where there's a lot of change, not just biological, so you do start to question where you go in terms of the future. It's a transitional period isn't it, with a lot of confusion, but also positive in terms of looking towards a different way of living, of not being a parent – well, always being a parent, but not always having the day to day looking after dependents.

Just thinking again about disentangling, I was taking to friends recently about how many men we know in their early to mid-fifties who have found it incredibly hard to cope with their work. They seem to get to a point in their jobs when they just can't sort of cope with it any longer. They might have been doing it for years and then suddenly, or maybe over a period of time, they feel they can't cope with it. Is it a thing about age? I know men go through hormonal change as well, obviously not in the same way. Perhaps it is something about doing the same job or being employed or having to be breadwinner? Maybe it's that pressure on them over a long period of time and then they get to a point when they feel that has to change, they can't sustain it? So, I just find it interesting that a lot of men that I've come across or know through other people, get to that point when they can't manage the work stresses they used to. I certainly feel like that. I've got to my mid-fifties and can't cope with some of the stresses that I used to and would have done maybe ten years ago. So, I don't think it's just a biological thing, losing oestrogen, or whatever.

SHENAGH

I think I feel even more of a woman being out the other side.

I was just thinking that my menopause was a relatively long time ago now so, it's not massively fresh in my memory, but I'm sure as I think it through and talk, things will come up.

My first memory is that my mother's menopause was quite quick and young as well. I don't know whether this is anything, but my mum's menopause – when her periods stopped – was not long after my father died. Whether it was the shock that took her into earlier menopause, I don't know. Emotionally she wasn't great, but then my mum's emotions were very, very high anyway. So, I remember her time, if you like, quite clearly, but I don't know whether that was coupled with her losing her husband and me losing my dad at the same time.

So, my menopause started probably when I was about … ah, you see, I'm struggling with when. I've been out the other side quite a time now, eight years, maybe more. Isn't that weird – it's the dim and distant past already?

My memories – well, physically, I suffered very much from night sweats and hot sweats. I remember that *very, very* vividly. I remember one time on the school run taking my son N who was at primary school at the time, so he was about ten. It was Year Six and I'm sixty now, so this is about ten years ago. Suddenly my face felt very, very hot and very, very red. I looked in the mirror and my face was completely *bright, bright* red. I looked like a tomato. I've never seen my face so strong and there was a sort of green tinge across the top of my lip. I turned to N and I said, 'Do I look red?' and he said, 'You need to look in the mirror, mum.' I thought I could *not* walk into school looking as I did, so he went in on his own. I think that was the most extreme visual experience.

I used to get really bad night sweats and my husband bought me – mainly so that he could get a more restful sleep (maybe that's a bit unfair) – a *Chillow Pillow* which worked really well. As the heat was rising up through my body it would then cool me down and I could get back off to sleep again. Therefore, this helped with the sleep deprivation as well, which, of course, had an impact on my mood the next day.

Concurrently, when I was in the menopause – I'm an actor – I had been introduced to something called Meisner: a theatrical approach by Sanford Meisner, which I was interested by, even fascinated by. I decided to enrol on a course for two years, a part-time course. What is Meisner about? In retrospect I think it's a bit wanky. It is about being completely open and completely free with what you're seeing, and naming it, both in other people and in yourself. I think it has its place, but I also think it can be very dangerous if in the wrong hands. I've used bits of it because anything you do you usually find something interesting to take from it, don't you? In principle, what Meisner is about is what you're feeling emotionally and how you perceive the other person to be feeling. So, in the midst of the emotional side of my menopause I was also doing Meisner. I've always joked that Meisner and menopause do not make very good bed fellows, because you're being told what somebody thinks they're seeing you're feeling, but *you* don't know yourself how you're feeling. You're having to accept what they say and repeat it back or give a response to it, being honest with yourself. I'm quite good, in some ways, about being honest about how I'm feeling, and I can actually be too direct. Then, everything emotional was much, much stronger. I'm an emotional person anyway which I didn't think helped, or maybe it did? I don't know. Anyway, I'm just explaining the timing of when I was in the menopause and what else was going on alongside it.

It's interesting, you know. I've got a husband and son – they didn't *seem* to be overly aware of anything being massively different. So, as I say, I am a heart-on-my-sleeve sort of person and I say what I think. I won't hurt anybody and will apologise if I've gone on too much or been a bit too cross. I would say though, at that period of time, my emotions were everywhere, all over the place. Out the other side now, I'm more *knowing* about what I'm saying and why I'm saying it, rather than it just being a reaction. And, as I say, I don't know whether the Meisner thing made those emotions and that expression of what I was feeling and thinking and doing more pronounced, or whether I would have been like that anyway. I don't know, but it's just quite an interesting observation.

I'm just thinking what I did health-wise? I went swimming, I did yoga and I walked. I just did herbal stuff, like evening primrose and other things like that. I certainly didn't want to go down the HRT route. It wasn't like the menopause was an issue in any form for me, it was just the nature of where I was at in my life as a woman. I didn't go and see the doctor. For me, it's a thing that you just do. I didn't feel any *less* of a woman at the time. I think I feel even *more* of a woman being out the other side.

When I chat to friends or see girl friends who are younger than me talking about where they're at now or expressing how they're feeling I think, 'Oh gosh, yes, I'm glad I'm not there anymore' and, actually, realise how quite straightforward my menopause was. I just saw it like most things with me, I'm afraid, 'Well, that's where you're at and that's what it is, and you just get on with it,' without being, you know, British stiff upper lip and all of that, because I'm not like that either.

There were a few of us at the same time doing it, so that always helps I think. Chatting to other friends who were in the same position, you feel like you're not on your own. I remember that being very helpful – sort of similar to if you're a parent chatting to other mums and comparing notes, sort of, 'Yes, thank god your child's doing the same as mine, or whatever.'

What else? I think I've been completely free from my early fifties and I'm sixty now. Fifty was fine. I didn't feel any sort of ageing thing, you know. How did I find it? Not empowering because I hate that word, and it's not even about being happy in your own skin. Well, you're in the skin that you're in aren't you, so that's what your body's doing and that's what you're about really.

When I was out of it, I did a theatre project called The Wardrobe project and that was a whole thing about how women felt about themselves menopausally or when they're through the other side of menopause. It was all to do with the clothes ones wears and how one presents oneself, and how women present themselves at a certain age. I think I've always not wanted to present myself as being anything other than what I was at that time, so I didn't feel any sort of loss of the *younger* Shenagh, and *older* Shenagh having to wear this kind of stuff now. It's just that you kind of adapt your clothes a bit – you might find that you can't quite get into those tight jeans like you used to be able to and that kind of thing, and flowy cardigans cover that tummy that has developed probably more since menopause or as you get older.

I think that's it – I've racked my brains enough now!

LORNA WRITES

Beyond the menopause

My menopause was some time ago, but the hormonal changes which take place during this process can affect you for the rest of your life, and I don't think most women are fully aware of this. I am going to explore some aspects of my life as a post-menopausal woman. This leads on to some thoughts about women's healthcare in general.

First of all, I want to consider some definitions.

What do we mean by the term menopause? Process or end point?

Some authorities still define the menopause as the point when all periods have ceased and talk about 'reaching the menopause'.

NHS Choices, for example, states: 'The menopause is when a woman stops having periods and is no longer able to get pregnant naturally.'

According to Wikipedia: '*Menopause*, also known as the *climacteric*, is the time in most women's lives when menstrual periods stop permanently, and they are no longer able to bear children... Medical professionals often define menopause as having occurred when a woman has not had any vaginal bleeding for a year.'

But in my experience, most women talk about 'going through the menopause' and use the word menopause to describe the *process* their bodies go through in the lead up to the final cessation of periods, rather than the *end point* of this process.

After all, once your periods have become sporadic and less and less frequent, you can only know with hindsight when they have actually ceased completely. It's not that useful to have a word that can only be used retrospectively, when what we need is a word to encompass all the changes which are happening to our bodies, as they happen.

Why does the terminology matter?

I strongly believe that good healthcare requires good communication between patient and health professional; doctors need to be aware of differences between common parlance and technical terms, and to check whether they and their patients are using the same words to mean the same things.

Doctors can confuse us when they tell us that we haven't reached the menopause, if by that they mean that our periods haven't stopped completely. If we tell a doctor we think we are menopausal, and they correct us and say we are 'peri menopausal', we can go away baffled, without getting the help we have asked for. The word 'peri menopausal' sounds like 'pre-menopausal', or even a bit like 'quasi-menopausal', as if the symptoms we are telling them about are not the genuine article.

Yet we are trying to describe the real changes which are already taking place. Final cessation of periods and an end to symptoms such as hot flushes, poor sleep, mood swings etc. would come as a blessed relief to most women (although probably not if you are experiencing an early menopause); but it is the years leading up to this cut-off point when we are most likely to be seeking help from a doctor.

Personally therefore, I usually refer to the menopause as the *process* which leads to the final cessation of menstruation, rather than the *end point*.

While we're on the subject of definitions, I have to confess I am bemused by the alternative term 'climacteric', (which I have never heard anyone use in everyday life) and which the online Oxford English Dictionary defines either as 'a critical period or event' or as 'the period of life when fertility and sexual activity are in decline; (in women) menopause.'

Leaving aside the suggestion that 'sexual activity' is in decline at this stage of life, which may or may not be the case, the implication of using this dramatic word 'climacteric' seems to be that the cessation of periods and the consequent loss of fertility are the most critical or significant events in a woman's life. For me at least, it was more of an anti-climax than a climax.

My menopause

Menopause itself wasn't a big deal for me. From the age of fifty, my periods got very irregular, both in frequency and intensity, and eventually stopped just before my fifty-fourth birthday. I had the odd hot flush, but I wasn't plagued with them, and certainly never woke up in the night bathed in sweat. (Neither am I still subject to hot flushes, unlike friends of mine who continue to have them in their late sixties. Has anyone ever mentioned that possibility to you before?)

At the time I was emerging from a very distressing few years which included a difficult relationship which came to a sticky end, and caring for my parents, both of whom were very ill in old age, until they died. To be honest, the menopause was the least of my worries.

Health wise at this time I was more concerned with the fact that I had been diagnosed with an underactive thyroid. My energy levels and blood test results kept fluctuating, and it took a while before the correct level of medication (thyroid hormone replacement) could be determined. I was repeatedly told the thyroid issue was nothing to do with the menopause, although everything I read about it seemed to suggest there was at the very least a strong correlation; it affects far more women than men and tends to start around the age of fifty. I never got to the bottom of the apparent connection between the two, but I learned to live with my hypothyroidism, an auto-immune condition which will be with me for the rest of my life.

Overall, however, as regards the menopause, I think I got off lightly. I had never suffered from excessively painful periods or from debilitating PMT, whereas at least one woman of my acquaintance who had endured maddening PMT for years, also experienced the menopause as mind-bendingly challenging. Is there any correlation, I wonder, between the level of discomfort women experience from their periods and the discomfort they go through at the menopause?

I had also fulfilled my desire to give birth (in the nick of time, just before I was forty) and was bringing up my young child, so I was not grieving for the imminent loss of my fertility. For friends of mine who wanted to have a baby, but were unable to do so, I have no doubt that menopause was much harder to bear.

Menopause – not the end of the story

I am now sixty-four, and the menopause seems a long time ago; periods and PMT even more remote.

But it turns out that I was not to be let off quite so lightly after all. I recently discovered that I now have an unpleasant condition called *Lichen sclerosus*. Never heard of it? Me neither! It appears that there is no end to the annoying or alarming things that can happen to our sexual and reproductive organs as we go through life.

Symptoms are: itching and soreness on and around the genitals; discoloration of the skin (it goes white in the affected area), which of course you wouldn't know about unless you were in the habit of examining your vulva regularly (something I am now advised to do); thinning and splitting of the skin, which is as painful as a paper cut in your nether regions; possible fusion of some of the affected tissue. Lichen sclerosus can affect other parts of the body, it can affect men as well as women, and it can also affect children, but this is rare: the majority of cases, so I understand, affect the genitals of post-menopausal women.

Lichen sclerosus is not infectious, nor sexually transmitted. It is yet another auto-immune condition, and, like the hypothyroidism, it is incurable, so I am stuck with it for good. The main symptoms can be managed, with a topical steroid cream and lavish use of emollient lotion. I was shocked to learn, though, on my second visit to the consultant, that some of the tissue around the vaginal opening has fused together, thus shrinking the orifice. The consultant has offered me minor surgery to separate the fused tissue to open it up again. Hmm. Something to think about there.

By the time it was diagnosed, I must have had it for ages. I had experienced soreness, itching, discomfort for a while but thought it was 'just one of those things' which I had to put up with. Vaseline seemed to help. I was puzzled by the stinging pain I experienced near my clitoris when I needed to push to do a poo. It felt just as if the skin was torn – which in fact it was – but somehow, I thought I must be imagining this because I couldn't explain it. Eventually I went to the doctor because I was waking up with an urgent need to pee many times each night. Tests for urinary tract infections were negative, and an abdominal scan revealed nothing untoward. My GP referred me to a consultant, who immediately diagnosed lichen sclerosus.

I could never have lasted as long as I did without getting it checked out by a doctor if I had been in an active sexual relationship. Gentle external stimulation would have been tricky; penetrative sex would have been torture. So, the reason I didn't find out what was happening sooner is because I hadn't had sex with a partner for a long time, and because I didn't know that this unnamed discomfort, I was experiencing was actually a thing. It's not an ailment most of us have heard of and it is one of those conditions, primarily or solely affecting women, which are not well recognised even amongst the medical profession.

Women are used to putting up with all sorts of pain and discomfort connected with our sexual and reproductive organs – it's all part of the curse of Eve – not to mention frequently being fobbed off when we know something is wrong but can't get doctors to investigate properly. So, we don't always go to the doctor when we should. Lichen sclerosus, ignored and untreated, may in rare cases (fewer than 5%) lead to vulval cancer – let alone ruining women's sex lives and relationships.

In the same way, we now know that many women have suffered for years with untreated endometriosis, sometimes leading to infertility, having been told that they just had heavy periods and shouldn't make such a fuss. '*Did you know it takes an average of 7.5 years for a woman to be diagnosed with endometriosis –*' asks the Royal College of Obstetricians and Gynaecologists on their blog, '– *a gynaecological condition surrounded by taboos, myths and a lack of awareness?*'

Recently there have also been newspaper reports about the failure of standard UTI tests to detect a hidden infection which has left thousands of women in chronic, disabling pain; not to mention the scandal of vaginal mesh implants, which have also left thousands of women in agony. In both cases it has taken years for the health service to take account of what women have been telling them, and to acknowledge these gross failures.

We are now learning that all over the world, women in pain wait longer for treatment and are less likely to be given effective painkillers than men. It really does seem that women are simply expected to put up with pain. Mustn't grumble!

Older women who find penetrative sex painful are usually told this is because hormonal changes have made the walls of the vagina thinner and dryer, and that the solution is to use lots of lube, and maybe an oestrogen cream. But now I wonder how many of these women actually have undiagnosed lichen sclerosus. Online forums are full of anguished accounts of women suffering for years, their sex lives in ribbons, before they received a correct diagnosis.

The consultant I saw said that many of his colleagues, even senior gynaecologists, were still insufficiently aware of lichen sclerosus; and it turns out I was lucky in that there is actually a vulval clinic at my local hospital – which is apparently quite rare – presided over by this well-informed and experienced consultant.

And for me personally? First of all, I have to say I am glad that it was recognised; I got a proper diagnosis and am now being treated and regularly reviewed. Of course, I feel fed up, not just with the pain and discomfort when it flares up, and the general nuisance of creams and lotions, but also because I have had to resign myself to the fact that this condition is with me for life.

More importantly, knowing that my beloved vulva is in such a sorry state has dashed my confidence and made me much more nervous about the prospect of starting a new sexual relationship if the opportunity arises.

What are the wider implications?

It is clear to me that women need much more information and proactive support, not just as we approach and experience the menopause, but also after the menopause.

These days, women are given at least basic advice and information at certain key points in their lives: most girls are taught what to expect when their periods start; advice is offered to (heterosexual) young women when they begin to be sexually active; information and support is offered to women who embark on pregnancy and motherhood; but where is the information pack, and the routine well-woman screening for every woman as she reaches middle age, and again as old age approaches?

Living with this wretched lichen sclerosus, and thinking about it for this piece, has reminded me forcibly of the excruciating pain I experienced the last time I had a cervical smear test, a few years ago. The nurse who carried out the test was totally incompetent, jammed the speculum in at the wrong angle, did not respond or stop when I screamed out, and left me with three lacerations in and around my vagina, confirmed by my GP when she examined me a few days later.

There is concern that fewer and fewer women are taking up the invitations to have regular smear tests. It is thought that this is because women feel 'embarrassed' when undergoing this procedure. What if it is not embarrassment, but previous experiences of pain, discomfort and insensitivity?

As a lesbian, I have always dreaded smear tests. I have always had to beg them to use the smallest possible speculum as the standard size is far too big. There seems to be an assumption that any mature woman must have been having frequent vigorous heterosexual intercourse for years and that this giant metal implement will slide in without any bother. (I have now realised, of course, that changes in my body since the menopause have made this procedure even more of an endurance test.)

Research some years ago found that lesbian and bisexual women were up to 10 times less likely to have had a cervical screening test in the past three years than heterosexual women. Clearly, there is something wrong with the way these tests are being administered which is putting so many of us off.

Lesbians have long complained that our particular experiences and health needs are not recognised or addressed by standard medical practice. Lesbians who took part in a survey conducted by the national LGB&T Partnership in 2016 reported that: clinicians tended to assume all their patients were heterosexual unless explicitly told otherwise; sometimes appeared uncomfortable when patients disclosed their sexual orientation; sometimes ignored this information even when it was clinically relevant; and sometimes gave misleading or incorrect health information to lesbians, based on myths and stereotypes.

But of course, it is not just lesbians, or lesbians of a certain age, who may find having a smear test painful and distressing. Like all health procedures, cervical smear tests should be conducted in a patient-centred way, finding out about our individual needs and circumstances before charging ahead.

Please don't assume we are all heterosexual. Please talk to us first and find out whether we are in a sexual relationship or not and if so, whether our sexual practice includes penetration. Do ask us about this before we are lying there half naked and spread-eagled upon the couch.

In conclusion

I think much greater attention needs to be given to women's health needs, beyond servicing our reproductive capacity. There needs to be more research into conditions which primarily affect women, better awareness and training for practitioners, and better public health education for women at every stage of their lives, and whatever path their life takes – recognising that lesbians have different health needs from heterosexual women, that older women's needs are different from younger women's needs, that some of us have children and some of us don't.

And don't forget that the menopause may signal the end of one phase of our life, but it is the beginning of the next phase, which brings with it its own challenges.

ACKNOWLEDGEMENTS

Thank you to …

Each of the remarkable women who share their stories – I cannot thank you enough for your honesty and courage.

Abigail Knight for sustaining conversations; Sallie Poppleton for a stream of *menopause alerts*; Lara Pawson for declaring, 'You've got to write the book, Caroline!'; Annie Johns for pondering ideas; Marcelle Hanselaar for playing with the title; Anouchka Grose for having confidence in the book; Anni McTavish for endless reassurance; Lucy Whitman for sharing professional expertise so generously.

And to Jayne Clavering, Alexandra Langley, Leigh Wilson, Nick Bertram, Gillian Murphy, Ginny Reddick, Angie Vollans, Toby Litt and Bharat Mistry who have each made a difference to this project.

Finally, to my cherished partner, Julian Grenier and my daughter, Maisie Vollans, for your staunch belief in this project. Thank you doesn't come close.

Also by Caroline Vollans

Wise Words: How Susan Isaacs Changed Parenting. Routledge (2017)

Celebrating Children's Learning (ed.) Routledge (2017)

What did you think?

If you would like to respond to *Menopause: 35 Women Speak* I would be interested to hear from you.

cvollans@gmail.com

twitter.com/CarolineVollans

Facebook.com/Caroline.Vollans.7

INDEX

Printed in Great Britain
by Amazon

87856036R00119